HYPERTENSION IN THE ELDERLY

KU-642-979

Developments in
Cardiovascular Medicine

VOLUME 157

The titles published in this series are listed at the end of this volume.

HYPERTENSION IN THE ELDERLY

Edited by

GASTONE LEONETTI
Istituto Scientifico, Ospedale San Luca, Milan, Italy

and

CESARE CUSPIDI
Centro di Fisiologia Clinica e Ipertensione, Ospedale Maggiore, Milan, Italy

MEDICAL LIBRARY
PEMBURY HOSPITAL
PEMBURY

Kluwer Academic Publishers
Dordrecht / Boston / London

*PM
95-118*

Library of Congress Cataloging-in-Publication Data

Hypertension in the elderly / edited by Gastone Leonetti and Cesare
.Cuspidi.
        p.   cm. -- (Developments in cardiovascular medicine ; v. 157)
    Includes index.
    ISBN 0-7923-2852-3 (HB : alk. paper)
    1. Hypertension in old age.   I. Leonetti, Gastone.   II. Cuspidi,
Cesare.   III. Series.
    [DNLM: 1. Heart Function Tests--in old age.   2. Heart-
-physiopathology.   3. Hypertension--in old age.   W1 DE997VME v. 157
1994 / WG 141.5.F9 H998 1994]
RC685.H8H787   1994
618.97'6132--dc20
DNLM/DLC
for Library of Congress   94-12005

ISBN: 0-7923-2852-3

Published by Kluwer Academic Publishers,
P.O. Box 17, 3300 AA Dordrecht, The Netherlands.

Kluwer Academic Publishers incorporates
the publishing programmes of
D. Reidel, Martinus Nijhoff, Dr W. Junk and MTP Press.

Sold and distributed in the U.S.A. and Canada
by Kluwer Academic Publishers,
101 Philip Drive, Norwell, MA 02061, U.S.A.

In all other countries, sold and distributed
by Kluwer Academic Publishers Group,
P.O. Box 322, 3300 AH Dordrecht, The Netherlands.

WG 340

*HYPERTENSION
AGED
WOODCLAMPS*

Printed on acid-free paper

All Rights Reserved
© 1994 Kluwer Academic Publishers
No part of the material protected by this copyright notice may be reproduced or utilized in any
form or by any means, electronic or mechanical, including photocopying, recording or by any
information storage and retrieval system, without written permission from the copyright owner.

Printed in The Netherlands

Contents

Foreword

GIUSEPPE MANCIA

From 1985 on, evidence has been accumulating that, in elderly hypertensive patients, blood pressure reduction by antihypertensive drugs is accompanied by a reduction in cardiovascular morbidity, mortality, and even total death rate. It has more recently been established that this is the case, not only for patients whose ages range between 60 and 70 years, but also for "old" elderly patients (i.e. patients aged above 70 years) and that the benefit of treatment included isolated systolic hypertension.

Given the high prevalence of hypertension in the elderly and the progressive senescence of the population, this means that antihypertensive drugs must be administered to a large and growing number of individuals, and that detailed information must be collected on all pathophysiological and clinical aspects of hypertension in old age in order for the choice of treatment to obtain a favourable efficacy/tolerance ratio in most subjects.

The present book aims at this goal with a series of chapters that cover some important issues. One issue concerns the hemodynamic changes and alterations of cardiovascular control mechanisms occurring with aging. Another issue deals with the way blood pressure should be measured in the elderly and with the role of ambulatory blood pressure monitoring (and, thus, blood pressure variability) in the diagnosis of hypertension and quantification of the antihypertensive response in old age. Some chapters are devoted to the effects of antihypertensive drugs and to the various treatment strategies available for the elderly. The benefit of antihypertensive treatment in the elderly is then reviewed by a separate description of the results of various intervention trails. All chapters are written by world-known experts in the field, which makes them informative and clear. I trust that the book will represent stimulating reading for all those interested in hypertension.

Gastone Leonetti and Cesare Cuspidi (eds), Hypertension in the Elderly, vii
© 1994 *Kluwer Academic Publishers. Printed in the Netherlands*

List of contributors

A. Amery, Hypertension Unit, Department of Internal Medicine, University
  Hospital Gasthuisberg, Herestraat 49, B-3000 Leuven, Belgium
Co-authors: R. van Hoof, L. Thijs, J. Staessen, R. Fagard, H. Celis and W.
  Birkenhäger

James B. Connelly, Senior Lecturer in Public Health Medicine, Academic
  Unit of Public Health Medicine, University of Leeds, 32 Hyde Terrace,
  Leeds LS2 9LN, U.K.

Cesare Cuspidi, Istituto Scientifico, Ospedale San Luca, Via Spagnoletto 3,
  I-20149 Milan, Italy

Peter W. de Leeuw, Department of Internal Medicine, University Hospital
  Maastricht, P.O. Box 5800, 6202 AZ Maastricht, The Netherlands
Co-author: Arie T.J. Lavrijssen

Tord Ekbom, Health Sciences Centre Dalby/Lund, Lund University, Helge-
  andsgatan 16, S-223 54 Lund, Sweden
Co-authors: Lars H. Lindholm, Lennart Hansson, Björn Dahlöf, Erland
  Linjer, Bengt Scherstén and Per-Olov Wester

Alberto U. Ferrari, Centro di Fisiologia Clinica e Ipertensione, Via F. Sforza
  35, I-20122 Milan, Italy

Gastone Leonetti, Istituto Scientifico, Ospedale San Luca, Via Spagnoletto
  3, I-20149 Milan, Italy

Giuseppe Mancia, Cattedra di Medicina Interna and 1° Divisione de Medicina Università di Milano and Ospedale S. Gerardo, Monza, Italy

Eoin O'Brien, The Blood Pressure Unit, Beaumont Hospital, Beaumont Road, P.O. Box 1297, Dublin 9, Ireland
Co-author: Kevin O'Malley

H. Mitchell Perry, Jr., Hypertension Unit, Washington University School of Medicine, Box 8048, 660 South Euclid Ave., St. Louis, MO 63110, U.S.A.
Co-authors: Kenneth G. Berge, M. Donald Blaufox, Barry R. Davis, Richard H. Grimm, Robert McDonald, Sara Pressel, Eleanor Schron, W. McFate Smith and Thomas M. Vogt

1. Changes in the cardiovascular system with aging

ALBERTO U. FERRARI

Introduction

Even in the absence of disease, aging brings about significant structural and functional changes in the cardiovascular system. Gaining knowledge of such changes is of great interest for clinicians, epidemiologists as well as basic scientists, but various difficulties hinder the way to achieve this goal.

First, in spite of the time-honored expression "Senectus ipsa morbus" (senescence is in itself a disease) coming to us from latin wisdom, a correct approach to the biology of aging, especially in human studies, is faced with the problem of separating alterations due to aging per se from those caused by diseases such as atherosclerosis, heart failure, diabetes mellitus, that are very common in the aged population in an either overt or concealed form. Second, although aging is commonly believed to promote a generalized decline in bodily functions, more and more evidence indicates that this is not always the case and that different functions may be differentially affected. In other words, age-dependent changes are so complex and selective that any general conclusion or extrapolation unsubstantiated by direct experimental assessment is likely to be in error and should not be attempted [1,2]. Third, on the opposite end of the spectrum of so-called "normalcy", studies adopting very restrictive entry criteria such as to only recruit individuals maintained under close health surveillance, dietary monitoring, sustained physical training, etc., may also reach conclusions not fully representative of the "average normal" elderly population.

Notwithstanding the methodological problems, evidence in this area is expanding so rapidly that any effort towards an exhaustive review would be unfeasible in the space of a few pages. This discussion will therefore restrict its focus on those age-related changes in the cardiovascular structure and function (including changes in humoral and renal factors) that are believed to more pronouncedly affect circulatory homeostasis.

Gastone Leonetti and Cesare Cuspidi (eds), Hypertension in the Elderly, 1–12
© 1994 *Kluwer Academic Publishers. Printed in the Netherlands*

Aging and the heart

The aging heart undergoes significant structural changes, with an increase in weight and some degree of left ventricular hypertrophy [3]. Fat content appears to increase whereas collagen content does not. Histologically, consistent although poorly understood alterations of the myocyte are lipofuchsin pigment deposition and basophilic degeneration. Unless heart disease co-exists, no age-related increase in resting left ventricular end-diastolic and end-systolic diameter is observed [4].

Functionally, resting heart rate and early diastolic filling rate decline slightly whereas resting indices of systolic performance such as ejection fraction, stroke volume or systolic work index are only minimally or not at all lowered. In contrast, more prominent changes characterize the cardiac responses to exercise. First of all, the exercise-induced rise in heart rate is less in aged as compared to young individuals. In addition, most indices of contractility increase less in the aged than in the young heart, so that in order to maintain adequate oxygen delivery to the exercising tissues the aging heart tends to more markedly augment its end-diastolic diameter, i.e. to more heavily engage the Starling mechanism in order to at least partially compensate for limited inotropic and chronotropic reserve. On the whole, the aging heart is said to cope with the challenge of exercise similarly to what a younger heart subjected to beta-adrenoceptor blockade would do [5,6]

Aging and the vascular system

Similar to the structural changes in the heart, some degree of age-related hypertrophy is also observed in the vascular media and intima (but not adventitia); arteries tend to become elongated and therefore tortuous; irregularities in the shape and size of endothelial cells, along with elastin fragmentation and calcification, are common changes [7].

Increased vascular stiffness is the universally observed and most important functional change associated with aging, although it is still debated whether this process develops because of aging per se or because of an increased load to the vessel walls [8,9]. Pulse wave velocity is increased in proportion to the arterial stiffening. A further point that is still to be clarified is whether the age-related changes in arterial mechanical properties are homogeneous throughout the arterial tree or there are qualitative and/or quantitative regional differences. In this regard, it is interesting to note that recent technological developments in ultrasound imaging make it possible to non-invasively and simultaneously assess conduit artery diameter and beat-to-beat arterial blood pressure, so that arterial compliance curves can be obtained over the systolic-to-diastolic pressure range in different segments of the arterial tree in vivo and in the absence of anesthesia [10]. Through this approach, an age-related reduction in arterial distensibility was generally confirmed [11], although preliminary evidence obtained by colleagues from our institute suggests that the compliance of the radial artery is not reduced and may rather tend to be increased in aged as compared to young subjects [12]. More evidence is clearly needed to draw reliable conclusions on this provocative possibility.

Due in part to large artery stiffness and in part to resistance arteriole hypertrophy, total peripheral resistance is also slightly augmented in advanced age [13]. The total and central blood volume are on the other hand reduced, and the effectiveness of regional hemodynamic regulation is partly impaired. Whether this depends on impaired autoregulatory mechanisms is unknown, but the endothelial function does appear to be reduced in advanced age, at least as far as the release of nitric oxide is concerned [14].

Aging and humoral cardiovascular control mechanisms

Aging is associated with disparate alterations of several humoral factors known to play important roles in cardiovascular regulation.

Plasma levels of catecholamines increase with age [15]: concerning norepinephrine this may be accounted for by a reduction in clearance as well as by an increase in spillover [16]. The latter would in turn be due to enhanced sympathetic nerve firing, as supported by various lines of evidence in both animals and humans (see below). As a consequence of the nervous overactivity, exaggerated catecholamine release and some degree of catecholamine depletion – that can be quantitatively assessed from a reduced tissue norepinephrine concentration – are also found in advanced age.

A further humoral pressor system that displays progressive age-related activation is the vasopressin system. Both basal and water deprivation-induced circulating vasopressin levels are higher in elderly as compared to young subjects: despite this, elderly subjects report less thirst during and lesser water intake after a water deprivation period [17].

At variance with the overactive sympatho-adrenergic and vasopressin systems, the renin–angiotensin system is depressed in old animals and humans. Supine plasma renin activity levels are diminished and so are the responses of the system to its activating physiological stimuli such as orthostasis, sodium depletion, hemorrage etc. [17]. It is likely that a hypofunctioning renin–angiotensin system contributes to the increased propensity of aged individuals to become dehydrated.

Finally, as a possible counterpart of the impaired renin–angiotensin system in the frame of a push-pull relationship, atrial natriuretic factor has been shown to be increased in advanced age. Again, this applies to both the unstimulated and the stimulated (via, e.g., a load of NaCl) circulating levels of the peptide [19].

The mechanisms underlying the humoral changes described above are far from being clarified due to the complex physiological interplay of various humoral factors to each other and to the central neural, baroreceptor reflex and the local circulatory control systems. For example, the age-related increase in vasopressin would on the one hand be in keeping with the concomitant increase in sympathetic activity because this peptide is known to facilitate sympathetic activity via a central and/or peripheral modulation. On the other hand, vasopressin is known to potentiate baroreceptor reflex influences [20], an effect that would entail reduced rather than enhanced sympathetic activity. A sympathetic facilitation is also exerted by angiotensin II that, however, is found to fall rather than to rise with aging. Also the age-related increase in ANF would be expected to restrain rather than to enhance sympathetic activity [21]. The reader can realize that any attempt to go into further detail on this topic would just be space-consuming and speculative in lack of adequate knowledge about which changes come first and which are, or are not, causally linked to each other during the aging process. Clearly, a tremendous research effort is needed in order to fill the present gaps and to consistently put together the pieces of this puzzle.

Aging and renal function

With aging, a 20–30% reduction of renal mass occurs, with the cortex being more markedly affected than the medulla. The nephron number is also reduced, with a preferential loss of juxtamedullary units having long loops of Henle and playing a crucial role in the urine concentration processes. In the glomeruli that survive, sclerosis and loss of capillary loops within the glomerular tuft and an augmented mesangial component are also generally observed [22,23].

Starting around the thirties, total renal blood flow declines about 10% per decade. The loss of cortical nephrons affects the intrarenal distribution of blood flow with a relative increase in medullary blood flow. The combination of the changes in the renal flow and of the age-related blood pressure elevation results in a rise in the calculated renal vascular resistance [24].

The renal function is reduced accordingly with the alterations described above: creatinine clearance linearly falls about 1% per year from the forties through the nineties. Lack of a concomitant rise in serum creatinine suggests that the production of this catabolyte also declines with age. The reduced glomerular filtration rate results in reduced elimination of some drugs cleared by the kidneys. The processes of urine acidification, concentration and dilution also lose part of their effectiveness with aging [25]. The ability of the aging kidney to produce erythropoietin and to metabolize hormones such as insulin, glucagon, calcitonin and parathyroid hormone have not yet been established.

Aging and cardiovascular homeostasis

Increased lability is the typical feature of the circulatory system in advanced age. Exaggerated blood pressure-falls are known to occur in response to assumption of the upright posture as well as under many other situations such as digestion, hemorrage, salt depletion, etc. [26]. Even independent of such specific circumstances, evaluation of overall 24-hour blood pressure variability may provide useful additional information on the age-related derangements in circulatory homeostasis. This was pursued in our laboratory by recording arterial blood pressure directly and continuously via a portable transducer-recorder device in a large group of subjects whose ages ranged widely. All subjects were ambulant inpatients so that their behaviour was standardized and therefore homogeneous. Data were analyzed beat-to-beat in order to obtain means and variabilities (expressed as the standard deviation of the mean as well as the percent variation coefficient) from the largest possible daily database. As shown in Figure 1, left panels, the older subjects had significantly larger blood pressure variability than the younger ones [27].

It is interesting to note that in the same subjects the increased blood pressure variability was accompanied by a reduced heart rate variability (Figure 1, right panels). Indeed, an age-related decline has been shown to characterize the cardiac chronotropic responses to a number of stimuli, mediated via sympathetic and/or vagal efferent fibres, including exercise, orthostasis, the Valsalva manoeuvre, cough, vasoactive drug injection, lower body negative pressure, etc. [28]. Thus along with an increase in blood pressure variability, aging brings about a change in the opposite direction in the variability of the heart rate. It is tempting to propose that, rather than chance, coexistence of the two phenomena reflects a causal link, namely that at least part of the increased blood pressure variability results from an impaired compensation for the moment-to-moment fluctuations in the total peripheral resistance as it can be exerted by reciprocal changes in the heart rate and hence in the cardiac output. This might not only apply to aging but also to disease conditions such as arterial hypertension [29], as well as to experimental conditions such as sino-aortic denervation [30] or cholinergic blockade [31], in all of which an increase in the blood pressure variability is associated with a reduction in heart rate variability. Evidence from an animal study supporting this concept is illustrated in Figure 2.

The mechanisms responsible for the impaired cardiovascular homeostasis with aging are complex and incompletely understood. A reduced effectiveness of cardiovascular reflex control has been convincingly documented, although it is increasingly recognized that the impairment is not uniform, and different reflex responses are differentially affected. Both human and animal experiments [32,33] indicate that within the arterial baroreflex the control of heart rate is markedly attenuated by aging whereas the control of efferent sympathetic activity and of blood pressure is much better preserved In a recent study on normotensive rats we could show that in the aged

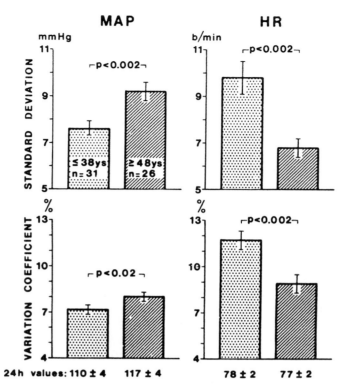

Figure 1. Variabilities of the mean arterial pressure (left) and of the heart rate (right) in subjects younger than 38 (dotted bars) and older than 48 (hatched bars) years. The older subjects had greater blood pressure and smaller heart rate variabilities than the younger ones, the difference being apparent by calculating variability either as standard deviation (top) or as variation coefficient (bottom).

animals the reflex chronotropic responses to vasoactive drug-induced changes in baroreceptor activity were about 50% less than in the younger animals (Figure 3), whereas in the same rats the peak pressor responses to bilateral common carotid artery occlusion were similar at all ages (Figure 4).

In human experiments employing microneurography, a technique by which efferent muscle sympathetic nerve activity can be directly recorded from the peroneal or brachial nerve, various authors including Grassi et al. in our institute, showed that the changes in sympathetic activity induced by stimulating and deactivating arterial baroreceptors by intravenous administration of phenylephrine and nitroglycerin, respectively, are not impaired in older as compared to younger subjects [34,35]. On the other hand, cardiopulmonary reflex influences seem to be rather extensively blunted by the aging process

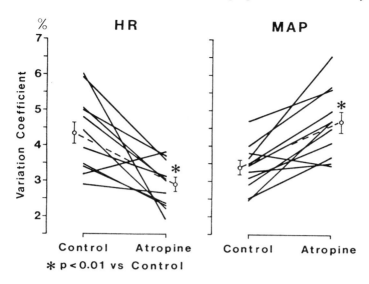

Figure 2. Effects of cholinergic blockade by atropine on the variabilities (computed as percent variation coefficients) of heart rate (HR) and of mean arterial pressure (MAP) in 11 individual rats (solid lines) and in the whole group of animals (open circles joined by dashed lines). Note that the reduction in heart rate variability produced by cholinergic blockade was accompanied by a marked increase in blood pressure variability.

although the experimental evidence in this area is much less extensive than for the arterial baroreflex system [36].

Evidence concerning the exact nature and location of the defect(s) responsible for the age-related decline in cardiovascular reflex control is also limited. The possibilities include various combinations of the following: loss and/or dysfunction of afferent baroreceptor elements, stiffness of the cardiac and vascular walls hosting the receptors, altered central neural processing of the afferent signal, and altered responsiveness of the effector organs to efferent autonomic influences.

The complexity of this area may be well exemplified by considering the numerous studies addressing the age-related changes in cardiac autonomic responsiveness. Various authors found the tachycardic responses to beta-receptor agonists to be reduced in aging subjects, probably because of a reduction in the number and/or affinity of beta-receptors in the sinus node [37,38]. Although this might contribute to the blunting of baroreflex modulation of the heart, it is to be emphasized that the baroreflex control of heart rate is mainly mediated by the vagus. In virtually total lack of information concerning cardiac parasympathetic responsiveness in advanced age, we [39] measured in senescent as compared to young rats the bradycardic responses to electrical stimulation of the distal end of the right vagus, the contralateral

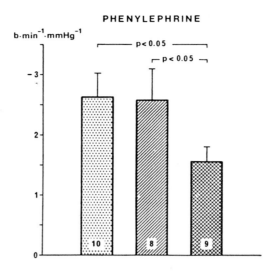

Figure 3. Effects of age on baroreceptor control of heart rate evaluated by the bradycardic and tachycardic responses to the rises and falls in blood pressure induced by in vivo phenylephrine and nitroprusside, respectively. Baroreflex sensitivity is expressed in beats per min per unit change in mean arterial pressure. Note the clearcut impairment of either reflex response in the old as compared to the adult and young rats.

vagus also being cut. This allowed the putative cardiac hyporesponsiveness to vagal stimuli to be directly evaluated in virtual open-loop conditions, i.e. in absence of confounding effects mediated by vagal afferents. Somewhat surprisingly, the old animals displayed enhanced rather than reduced brady-

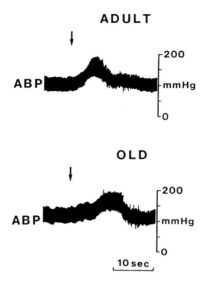

Figure 4. Examples from one adult and one old conscious rat showing the pressor response to bilateral common carotid artery occlusion (onset of the manoeuvre indicated by arrow). Note the slower time course but the unchanged magnitude of the blood pressure rise in the old as compared to the younger rat.

cardic responses to the whole range of electrical stimulation frequencies (Figure 5), indicating that at least in the normotensive rat, cardiac vagal responsiveness is not necessarily involved in the impairment of the baroreceptor–heart rate reflex and that the defective portion of the reflex is to be looked for elsewhere. To provide a comprehensive explanation of the experimental findings in this area, we speculatively propose that aging is normally associated with opposite changes in the vagal and sympathetic control of the heart: sympathetic activity would increase [35,40] whereas vagal activity would diminish [41,42]. Adaptive changes in cardiac autonomic receptors would promote down-regulation and up-regulation of cardiac adrenergic and cholinergic receptors, respectively [37,43]. Needless to say, also in this area much more experimental evidence is warranted to confirm or disprove the picture outlined above.

Conclusions

In conclusion, recent research advances outlined a complex and diversified picture of age-associated cardiovascular alterations, the most important of which are: – a reduced resting and effort cardiac output, possibly as a consequence of partially impaired systolic and diastolic function; – a slight

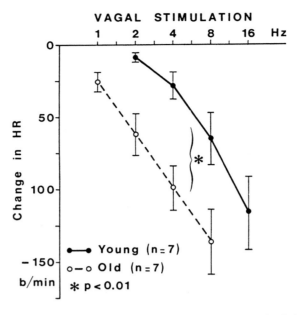

Figure 5. Mean (±SEM) bradycardic responses to graded electrical stimulation of the right efferent vagus from 1–16 Hz in anesthetized vagotomized rats of young and old age. The old animals 3- to 4-fold larger responses than the young ones.

increase in left ventricular mass and in total peripheral resistance; – a reduction in tissue perfusion and in the functional reserve of many organs and systems; – a relative hypovolemia and a depression of the renin-angiotensin system; – an impairment of cardiopulmonary and to a lesser extent of arterial baroreceptor reflexes, i.e. of the two major reflex systems controlling blood pressure and blood volume as well as water and sodium handling by the kidney; – an imbalance of cardiovascular autonomic drive with increased sympathetic and reduced parasympathetic activity; – a deranged circulatory homeostasis resulting in enhanced spontaneous blood pressure variability and exaggerated blood pressure falls in response to various stimuli such as orthostasis, food ingestion and sodium restriction.

Future research will have to elucidate the so far poorly understood mechanisms (e.g., central neural cardiovascular control, newer humoral substances, endothelial factors, etc.) underlying the age-related alterations of the cardiovascular system as well as to address the effects of aging on organs and functions that may importantly affect the circulation, but have been little or not at all explored.

References

1. Lipsitz LA. Abnormalities in blood pressure homeostasis associated with aging and hyper-

tension. In: Horan MJ, Steinberg GM, Dunbar JB, Hadley EC, editors. Blood Pressure Regulation and Aging. New York: Biomedical Information Corporation 1986: 201–11.

2. Ferrari AU, Grassi G, Mancia G. Alterations in reflex control of the circulation associated with aging. In: Amery A, Staessen J, editors. Handbook of Hypertension, volume 12 (Hypertension in the elderly). Amsterdam: Elsevier Science Publishers 1989: 39–50.

3. Miller TR, Grossman SJ, Schechtmann KB, Biello DR, Ludbrook PA, Ehsani AA. Left ventricular diastolic filling and its association with age. Am J Cardiol 1986; **58**: 531–5.

4. Rodeheffer RJ, Gerstenblith G, Becker LC, Fleg JL, Weistfeld ML, Lakatta EG. Exercise cardiac output is maintained with advancing age in healthy human subjects: cardiac dilatation and increased stroke volume compensate for diminished heart rate. Circulation 1984; **69**: 203–13.

5. Julius S, Antoon A, Witlock LS, Conway J. Influence of age on the hemodynamic response to exercise. Circulation 1976; **36**: 222–30.

6. Lakatta EG. Cardiovascular reserve and aging. In: Horan MJ, Steinberg GM, Dunbar JB, Hadley EC, editors. Blood Pressure Regulation and Aging. Biomedical Information Corporation 1986: 51–78.

7. Stemermann MB, Weinstein R, Rowe JW, et al. Vascular smooth muscle cell growth kinetics in vivo in aged rats. Proc Natl Acad Sci USA 1982; **79**: 3863–6.

8. Roach MR, Burton AC. The effect of age on the elasticity of human iliac arteries. Can J Biochem Physiol 1959; **37**: 557–70.

9. Roy CS. The elastic properties of the arterial wall. J Physiol 1981; **3**: 125–59.

10. Meiste JJ, Tardy Y, Stergiopulos N, Hayoz D, Brunner HR, Etienne JD. Non-invasive method for the assessment of non-linear elastic properties and stress of forearm arteries in vivo. J Hypertens 1992; **10**(Suppl 6): s23–s26.

11. Boutouryrie P, Lauren S, Benetos A, Girerd XJ, Hoeks APG, Safar ME. Opposing effects of ageing on distal and proximal large arteries in hypertensives. J Hypertens 1992; **10**(suppl 6): s87–s91.

12. Giannattasio C, Mancia G. Personal communication.

13. Soltis EE, Webb RC, Bohr DF. The vasculature in hypertension and aging. In: Horan MJ, Steinberg GM, Dunbar JB, Hadley EC, editors. Blood Pressure Regulation and Aging. New York: Biomedical Information Corporation 1986: 5141–55.

14. Iwama I, Kato T, Muramatsu M, et al. Correlation with blood pressure of the acetylcholine-induced endothelium-derived contracting factor in the rat aorta. Hypertension 1992; **19**: 326–32.

15. Ziegler MG, Lake CR, Kopin IJ. Plasma noradrenaline increases with age. Nature 1976; **261**: 333–35.

16. Esler M, Skews H, Leonard P, et al. Age-dependence of noradrenaline kinetics in normal subjects. Cli Sci 1981; **60**: 217–9.

17. Helderman JH, Vestal RE, Rowe JW, Tobin JD, Andres R, Robertson GL. The response of arginine vasopressin to intravenous ethanol and hypertonic saline in man: the impact of aging. J Gerontol 1978; **33**: 39–47.

18. Hayduk K, Krause DK, Kaufman W, Huenges R, Schillmoller U, Unbehaun B. Age-dependent changes of plasma renin concentration in humans. Cli Sci 1973; **45**: 273s–278s.

19. MacKnight JA, Roberts J, Sheridan B, Atkins AB. Relationship between basal and sodium-stimulated plasma atrial natriuretic factor, age, sex and blood pressure in normal man. J Human Hypertension 1989; **3**: 157–63.

20. Undesser KP, Hasser EM, Haywood JR, Johnson AK, Bishop VS. Interactions of vasopressin with the area postrema in arterial baroreflex function in conscious rabbits. Cir Res 1985; **56**: 410–7.

21. Ferrari AU, Daffonchio A, Sala NC, Gerosa S, Mancia G. Atrial natriuretic factor and arterial baroreceptor reflexes in unanesthetized rats. Hypertension 1990; **15**: 162–7.

22. Dunnil MS, Halley W. Some observations on the quantitative anatomy of the kidney. J Pathol 1973; **110**: 113–21.

23. Davies DF, Shock NW. Age changes in glomerular filtration rate, effective renal plasma flow, and tubular excretory capacity in adult males. J Clin Invest 1950; **29**: 496–507.

24. Tauchi H, Tsuboi K, Okutomi J. Age changes in the human kidney of different races. Gerontologia 1971; **17**: 87–97.
25. Hilton JG, Goodbody MF Jr, Kruiesi OR. The effect of prolonged administration of NH$_4$Cl on the blood acid-base equilibria of geriatric subjects. J Am Ger Soc 1955; **3**: 697–703.
26. Ferrari AU. Age-related modifications in neural cardiovascular control. Aging Clin Exp Res 1992; **4**: 183–95.
27. Mancia G, Ferrari A, Gregorini L, et al. Blood pressure and heart rate variabilities in normotensive and hypertensive human beings. Circ Res 1983; **53**: 96–104.
28. Kalbfleisch JH, Reinke JA, Porth CJ, Ebert TG, Smith JJ. Effect of age on circulatory response to postural and Valsalva tests. Proc Soc Exp Biol Med 1977; **156**: 100–3.
29. Conway J, Boon N, Davies C, Jerres JV, Sleight P. Neural and humoral mechanisms involved in blood pressure variability. J Hypertense 1984; **2**: 203–8.
30. Bertinieri G, Cavallazzi A, Jaslitz L, Ramirez AJ, DiRienzo M, Mancia G. Differential control of blood pressure and heart rate by carotid and aortic baroreceptors in unanesthetized cats. J Hypertens 1987; **5**: 55–6
31. Ferrari AU, Daffonchio A, Albergati F, Mancia G. Inverse relationship between heart rate and blood pressure variabilities in rats. Hypertension 1987; **10**: 533–7.
32. Parati G, Frattola A, Castiglioni P, DiRienzo M, Ulian L, Mancia G. Invecchiamento e sensibilita del barroriflesso: studio mediante analisi delle variazioni di pressione arteriosa e di frequenza cardiaca nelle 24 ore. X Congr Naz Soc It Ipertens Arteriosa, 1993: **32** (Abstract).
33. Ferrari AU, Daffonchio A, Albergati F, Mancia G. Differential effects of aging on the heart rate and blood pressure influences of arterial baroreceptors in awake rats. J Hypertension 1991; **9**: 615–21.
34. Ebert TJ, Morgan BJ, Barney JA, Denahan T, Smith JJ. Effects of aging on baroreflex regulation of sympathetic activity in humans. Am J Physiol 1992; **263**: H798–H803.
35. Grassi G, Seravalle G, Cattaneo BM, Lanfranchi A, Bolla GB, Mancia G. Modificazioni nervose simpatiche e controllo riflesso del circolo nell'anziano. X Congr Naz Soc It Ipertens Arteriosa, 1993: **86** (Abstract).
36. Cleroux J, Giannattasio C, Bolla GB, et al. Decreased cardiopulmonary reflexes with aging in normotensive humans. Am J Physiol 1989; **257**: H961–H968.
37. Van Brummelen P, Buhler FR, Kiowski W, Amann FW. Age-related decrease in cardiac and peripheral vascular responsiveness to isoprenaline: studies in normal subjects. Cli Sci 1981: **60**: 571–7.
38. Feldman RD, Limbird LE, Nadeau J. Alterations in leukocyte beta-receptor affinity with aging. N Engl J Med 1984; **310**: 815–9.
39. Ferrari AU, Daffonchio A, Gerosa S, Mancia G. Alterations in cardiac parasympathetic function in aged rats. Am J Physiol 1991; **260**: H647–H649.
40. Hajduczok G, Chapleau MW, Johnson SL, Abboud FM. Increase in sympathetic activity with age. Role of impairment of arterial baroreflexes. Am J Physiol 1991; **260**: H1113–H1120.
41. Alicandri C, Boni E, Fariello R, et al. Parasympathetic control of heart rate and age in essential hypertensive patients. J Hypertens 1987; **5**: s345–s347.
42. Dauchot P, Gravenstein JS. Effects of atropine on the electrocardiogram in different age groups. Clin Pharmacol Ther 1971; **12**: 274–80.
43. Ferrari AU, Daffonchio A, Franzelli C, Mancia G. Cardiac parasympathetic hyperresponsiveness in spontaneously hypertensive rats. Hypertension 1992; **19**: 653–7.

2. Blood pressure measurement in the elderly with special reference to ambulatory blood pressure measurement

EOIN O'BRIEN and KEVIN O'MALLEY

Introduction

Elderly patients with hypertension constitute a group within the hypertensive population deserving of special attention. Not alone are the elderly susceptible to the adverse effects of blood pressure-lowering drugs [1], but blood pressure measurement in the elderly presents particular problems which, if not recognised, must lead inevitably to incorrect diagnosis and unnecessary treatment [2]. The purpose of this paper is to put the problems of blood pressure measurement in the elderly into perspective and to assess the role of ambulatory blood pressure measurement (ABPM) in achieving a more accurate profile of blood pressure behaviour.

The prevalence of hypertension increases with age [3] and hypertension is a major risk for the development of cardiovascular disease in elderly patients [4]. Furthermore, the European Working Party on Hypertension in the Elderly has shown that antihypertensive therapy is beneficial in reducing the cardiovascular complications of hypertension in elderly patients [5]. It has been estimated that more than 40% of elderly hypertensive patients receive regular antihypertensive medication [6], and recently the accuracy of diagnosis which destines so many elderly people to life-long medication has been questioned [2, 7].

The vascular, structural and functional factors that lead to a tendency for elderly patients to develop predominantly systolic hypertension have been reviewed by Messerli and colleagues [2]. The results of the SHEP Study indicate considerable benefit in reducing isolated systolic hypertension in the elderly [8] but these results may not be applicable to all populations and the Syst-Eur study, which embodies in its design a side-project on 24-hour ABPM, is presently being conducted in Europe [9]. Until recently, therefore, the information on which we base therapeutic and management decisions in elderly patients with hypertension has derived from conventional blood pres-

Gastone Leonetti and Cesare Cuspidi (eds), Hypertension in the Elderly, 13–25
© 1994 *Kluwer Academic Publishers. Printed in the Netherlands*

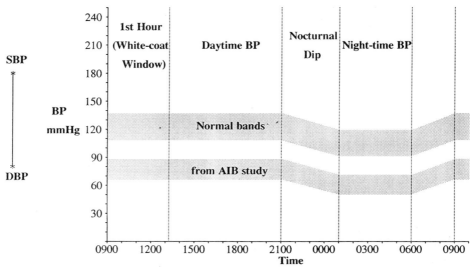

Figure 1. Scheme for presentation of data: OBP = Office Blood Pressure; SBP = Systolic Blood Pressure; DBP = Diastolic Blood Pressue; The 24-hour period is divided into four windows – the white coat window during the first hour of recording when blood pressure may be elevated due to the white coat effect; the day time window; the retiring window when the blood pressure may dip and the night-time window. The mean blood pressures for each of these windows is printed across the top of the plot and the percentage nocturnal dip in blood pressure. The shaded bands indicate the upper and lower limits of blood pressure as derived from the Allied Irish Bank Study (O'Brien E, Murphy J, Tyndall A, et al. Twenty-four-hour ambulatory blood pressure in men and women aged 17–80 years. The Allied Irish Bank Study. J Hypertens 1991; **9**: 255–360).

sure measurement which may be influenced by factors common to all age groups with hypertension, such as the white coat effect and hypotension and certain factors peculiar to the elderly, such as isolated systolic hypertension and pseudohypertension [2].

Problems of blood pressure measurement common to all age groups but possibly of particular relevance in the elderly

White coat hypertension

White coat hypertension, the phenomenon whereby office blood pressures are elevated but may fall to normal levels during ABPM, is common, affect-

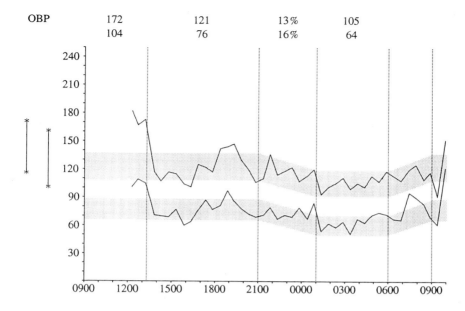

Figure 2. White coat hypertension.

ing some 20% of patients with hypertension [10]. In discussing white coat hypertension, it is important to establish definitions so as to avoid confusion. We propose that the term *white coat hypertension* should be reserved for those patients who exhibit elevated office blood pressures which settle within a short time to give normal daytime mean blood pressure (Figure 2) and that the term *white coat effect* should be reserved for those patients who exhibit elevated office blood pressures which reduce with ABPM but do not lower the mean daytime blood pressure to normal (Figure 3).

Blood pressure variability is increased in the elderly [2] and there is some evidence that both white coat hypertension and the white coat effect are more prevalent in older subjects [11, 14] thus raising the important question as to how much reliance can be placed on conventional office blood pressure measurement in the diagnosis of hypertension in the elderly [15]. In fact, if we accept that the most effective method for diagnosing white coat hypertension and white coat effect in the younger hypertensive is by ABPM, then the argument in favour of applying the technique to the elderly becomes all the more compelling if the prevalence of the white coat phenomenon is more common in this age group. The case becomes all the more persuasive when consideration is given to the issue of protecting elderly patients from unnecessary or excessive antihypertensive medication while being conscious of not withholding treatment that may have its greatest benefit in this age group. It is our practice to perform 24-hour ABPM in all elderly patients to exclude

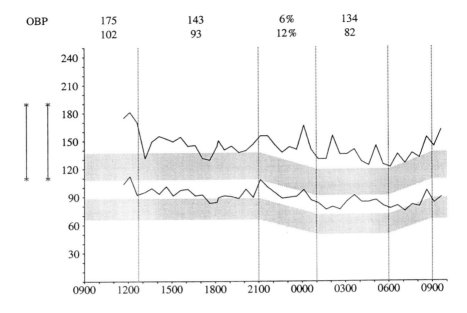

Figure 3. White coat effect.

white coat responders, while accepting that the white coat response may not be a normal phenomenon but one which merits continuing observation but not necessarily antihypertensive medication.

Assessment of nocturnal blood pressure

There is now growing evidence that hypertensive patients whose nocturnal blood pressure decline – so-called 'dippers' – have less cardiovascular damage and consequent risk than the minority of patients whose blood pressure fails to reduce at night – 'non-dippers' [16–19]. There is as yet little evidence to suggest that blood pressure patterns in elderly patients differ greatly during sleep from younger age groups [20], but as the quality of sleep alters with advancing years it may not be surprising if differences between age groups emerge as more data become available.

Perhaps of greater relevance in the aged is the possibility that excessive lowering of nocturnal blood pressure by critically altering perfusion of vital organs may predispose to cardiac and cerebral ischaemic events [21, 22]. It is reasonable to assume that the elderly, in whom cardiovascular haemodynamics are often compromised, are more susceptible to cerebrovascular events consequent upon excessive reduction of nocturnal blood pressure resulting from excessive antihypertensive medication. Such an occurrence would be especially likely in elderly hypertensive patients who exhibit a

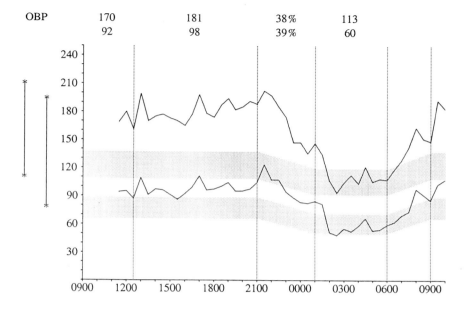

Figure 4. Daytime hypertension with large nocturnal dipping pattern.

pronounced nocturnal dipping pattern (Figure 4). Nocturnal blood pressure can only be characterised by 24-hour ABPM which should be performed in elderly patients so as to avoid excessive blood pressure lowering at night.

Hypotension

Hypotension, particularly related to posture, may affect all age groups [23] but is particularly common in the elderly, occurring in 10% of otherwise healthy elderly hypertensive subjects [24]. Symptomatic hypotension is particularly prevalent among the elderly in whom autonomic dysfunction is common [25]. Using conventional measurement these patients may appear hypertensive but 24 hour ABPM may show periods of sustained hypotension (Figure 5). Clearly the administration of antihypertensive medication to such patients could be disadvantageous and ABPM is proving a valuable technique for assessing such patients [25].

The elderly are also prone to another hypotensive phenomenon – post-prandial hypotension. It is often not recognised how common this phenomenon is in the elderly [2]. Blood pressure may fall by as much as 25 mmHg in response to a meal in elderly institutionalised patients [26]. The phenomenon of post-prandial hypotension can be demonstrated by ABPM, thus identifying an important subgroup of elderly hypertensive patients who require especial management [25].

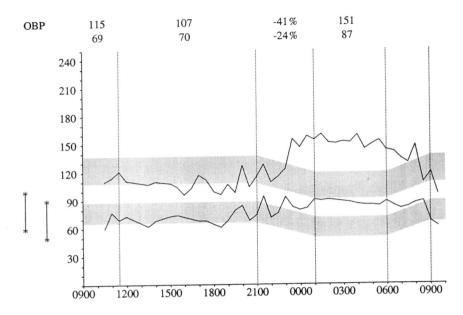

Figurer 5. Autonomic failure.

General aspects of blood pressure measurement

Blood pressure measurement in the elderly should not differ in principle from that in the population as a whole and standard recommendations, such as those of the British Hypertension Society should be carefully followed [27]. However, three aspects of blood pressure measurement should be given especial consideration in the elderly. First, selection of the correct bladder is important for both conventional measurement and ABPM. It is important to avoid undercuffing which may lead to over-estimation of blood pressure, but in the elderly lean arms are not uncommon and it is also important to avoid overcuffing with the attendant risk of under-estimating blood pressure [28]. Secondly, the occurrence of an auscultatory gap may be more common in the elderly simply because the level of systolic blood pressure tends to be higher in this age group and palpation of the radial pulse before auscultation is particularly important so as to avoid underestimating systolic blood pressure [2]. Finally, for reasons already referred to, it is important in the elderly to measure blood pressure in the lying, standing and sitting positions so as to detect postural hypotension which may be particularly common in this age group.

Problems of blood pressure measurement which tend to be occur only in the elderly

Isolated systolic hypertension

Isolated systolic hypertension is a common condition of the elderly occurring in 8% of people in the age stratum 60–69 years and rising to 22% for those aged 80 years or older [8]. These percentage estimates translate into a daunting reality that nearly 4 million Americans aged 60 and older have isolated systolic hypertension [8] and are likely to be considered candidates for antihypertensive medication. However, it must be borne in mind that all such statistics derive from data based on conventional blood pressure measurement. While there is no denying the risk of isolated systolic hypertension [3], a case can perhaps be made along the lines that while it is likely that benefit will be derived from the treatment of isolated hypertension [8], not all who receive such treatment need it. Is there any evidence to suggest that such an assertion can be upheld?

In 1990, Silagy and colleagues demonstrated that in a small number of elderly subjects with isolated systolic hypertension mean ambulatory blood pressures were consistent with that diagnosis for only 8% of the daytime period [13]. In another study Cox and colleagues also showed a marked discrepancy between clinic and daytime pressures in patients with isolated systolic hypertension with the former being some 27 mmHg higher than ambulant pressures. These results have been confirmed in the preliminary analysis of the ambulatory side-project of the Syst-Eur Study [29]. These findings suggest that isolated systolic hypertension is not always a sustained phenomenon and that in many patients the observed rise in office pressure is a manifestation of an alerting reaction [30]. We have, therefore, two forms of isolated systolic hypertension on ABPM – 'sustained' isolated systolic hypertension and 'transient' isolated systolic hypertension (Figures 6, 7). It may be postulated that antihypertensive medication could be targeted particularly at those elderly patients with sustained isolated hypertension on ABPM. However, before making such a recommendation, it would be necessary to know if cardiovascular risk was predicted more accurately by ABPM than by conventional measurement.

An increasing number of studies have demonstrated that ambulatory pressures correlate more closely than clinic pressures with several different indices of target organ damage [18, 19, 31]. In a preliminary analysis of ambulatory measurements of blood pressure carried out on 46 patients in the run-in phase of the ambulatory monitoring side-project of the Syst-Eur study, ECG voltage criteria for left ventricular hypertrophy correlated more with ABPM than with office blood pressure, suggesting that ambulatory measurement is a better predictor of left ventricular hypertrophy than clinic measurement in elderly patients with hypertension [32, 33]. It is anticipated that the Syst-Eur

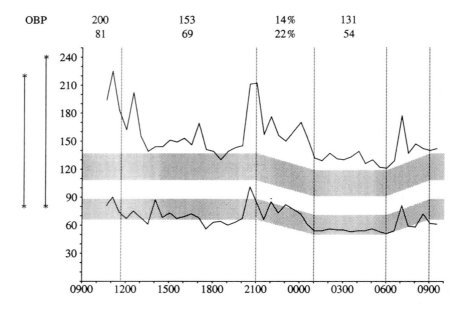

Figure 6. 'Sustained' isolated systolic hypertension.

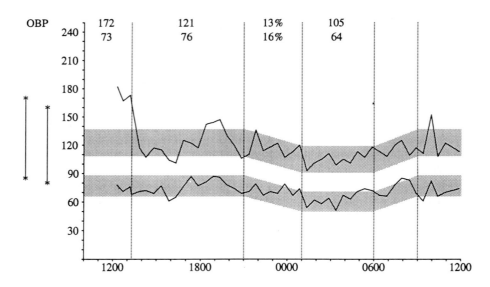

Figure 7. 'Transient' isolated systolic hypertension.

study should provide the answer to this important question before long. Until such information becomes available, ABPM should be used in elderly patients with isolated systolic hypertension to identify those with sustained elevation of systolic blood pressure who may require drug treatment and those in whom elevation of systolic pressure is not sustained, in whom the decision to treat may be influenced by additional factors, such as the presence of end organ involvement.

Pseudohypertension

In 1978, Spence and colleagues described a condition in some elderly patients with apparent hypertension diagnosed by conventionally measured blood pressure in whom directly measured intra-arterial blood pressure was normal [34]. Messerli and his colleagues proposed distinguishing between true hypertension and 'pseudohypertension' in these patients by the use of Osler's manoeuvre [35]. In this manoeuvre the blood pressure cuff is inflated above systolic pressure and if the artery distal to the cuff is palpable the sign is present. Osler used the sign to detect 'sclerosis' of the vessel wall [36]. Having classified hypertension thus, Messerli et al. went on to show that arterial compliance was lower in Osler-positive patients and that decreased compliance correlated with the difference between direct and indirect blood pressure indicating that the stiffer the artery the greater the degree of 'pseudohypertension' [35].

A number of important questions, however, remain to be addressed. To what extent does the presence of a positive Osler sign predict 'pseudohypertension'? While the direct–indirect difference correlates with decreased compliance the percentage of variance attributable to decreased compliance is small at about 26% in normotensive elderly people [35, 37]. Furthermore, there are few data on the prevalence of the sign in hypertension, and there may well be poor concordance between observers in eliciting it [38]. Finally, the sign is frequently present in those who are normotensive on the basis of cuff blood pressure [39].

We have examined the accuracy of indirect blood pressure measurement in elderly hypertensives and compared it with that in younger patients [40]. Indirect measurement underestimated direct systolic pressure by 4.4 mmHg in the elderly and 7.0 mmHg in the young and overestimated diastolic blood pressure by 9.2 mmHg and 10.4 mmHg, respectively. This study was conducted in consecutive patients presenting in our blood pressure clinic and were reasonably representative of ambulant hypertensive patients referred to such a clinic. Our findings led us to conclude that the standard technique for blood pressure measurement with a mercury sphygmomanometer is as accurate in the elderly as in young patients in general. However, that is not to say that there are not some elderly hypertensive patients, prevalence unknown, who have a large disparity between direct and indirect blood pressure measure-

ment and in such circumstances conventional sphygmomanometry may over-
estimate both systolic and diastolic blood pressure.

'Pseudohypertension' is probably not a good term as in many such cases
hypertension is correctly diagnosed but it is the severity which is overestimated; a better term might be 'inappropriate hypertension'. Some patients
will, however, be misdiagnosed as hypertensive because their intra-arterial
pressure is 'normal' while the cuff pressure is in the hypertensive range.
Here the term 'pseudohypertension' is apposite [41].

*ABPM in guiding the selection of appropriate blood pressure lowering drugs
for the elderly*

ABPM may prove to be a valuable technique in guiding the prescribing
physician in the choice of antihypertensive drug most suited for an individual
patient regardless of age, though this role for ABPM in clinical practice
awaits further study [42]. In this regard, however, ABPM may prove to be
especially helpful in the elderly [7, 43]. The technique permits determination
of those elderly patients in whom office blood pressure is elevated due to
white coat hypertension or the white coat effect and treatment can be selected
for those patients with sustained hypertension on ABPM. Moreover, ABPM
provides an assessment of the entire 24-hour profile thereby allowing the
determination of the dipper status and the selection of a short acting drug
for those elderly patients with marked nocturnal reduction of blood pressure,
or alternatively, selection of a longer acting drug for those with a non-dipping
nocturnal pattern. Patients with autonomic failure and postural hypotension
can be identified and the symptoms of hypotension avoided by judicious
prescribing. Finally, using ABPM it is possible to determine if symptoms
attributed to the blood pressure lowering effect of drugs are due to hypotension.

Are blood pressure measuring devices less accurate in the elderly?

If conventional blood pressure measurement presents a problem in the elderly, it is not unreasonable to assume that automated and semi-automated
devices will also have difficulty in recording accurate blood pressure measurements. In fact, the British Hypertension Society (BHS), in its revised protocol
for validating blood pressure measuring systems, has devoted a sub-section
to validation of devices in the elderly [45]. This recommendation is based
on evidence that age may affect device accuracy [46], and we have shown
that device accuracy worsens with increasing blood pressure levels [47]. In
choosing an ambulatory system consideration must be given to the accuracy
of the device in measuring the levels of blood pressure likely to be encountered in the subjects in whom ambulatory blood pressure is being measured.
As high blood pressures, especially for systolic blood pressure, may be
encountered in the elderly careful consideration should be given to the

available validation data before purchasing expensive ambulatory systems. On the basis of our analysis of six ambulatory devices according to pressure levels the CH-Druck and SpaceLabs 90207 were the most accurate though they were not as accurate in the higher pressure ranges [47]. However, the evidence available on device accuracy in the elderly is limited and it is imperative to conduct further validation studies in older age groups according to the revised BHS protocol [44].

Conclusion

Elderly patients with hypertension present a challenge to the diagnostic and management skills of their physician. On the one hand there is the important issue of diagnosis. Does the patient have hypertension or not? Because of the white coat phenomenon and the fact that isolated systolic hypertension appears only to be an office phenomenon in many patients makes ABPM an essential investigation for the accurate diagnosis of hypertension in the elderly. There are then idiosyncratic aspects of blood pressure behaviour in the elderly among which are the phenomenon of isolated systolic hypertension, increased variability of blood pressure and autonomic dysfunction each of which can be categorised more accurately with ABPM than with conventional measurement. When it comes to treating the elderly patient with hypertension ABPM can prove a useful adjunct to conventional measurement. It permits selection of the most appropriate blood pressure lowering drug for the individual patient taking into account the pattern of blood pressure throughout the day and night and thereby avoiding administration of excessive drug during periods of endogenous blood pressure lowering, such as during sleep. In assessing the common manifestations of hypotension in the elderly ABPM permits the association of symptoms with actual blood pressure levels. In concluding that ABPM should now be used in the assessment of elderly patients with apparent hypertension on conventional measurement the need to select carefully devices of proven accuracy is emphasised.

Finally, the relationship of ABPM to end organ damage is the subject of on-going studies which should be a reminder that blood pressure whether measured by conventional techniques or ABPM is only one aspect of the elderly patient's cardiovascular profile. Assessing target organ disease by echocardiography and an increasing range of investigations permits an assessment of the impact of blood pressure on the cardiovascular system which is likely to determine ultimately the outcome.

Acknowledgements

Support from the Charitabie Infirmary Charitable Trust, the Royal College of Surgeons in Ireland and Beaumont Hospital is acknowledged with gratitude.

References

1. Lamy P. Potential adverse effects of antihypertensive drugs in the elderly. J Hypertens 1988; **6** (Suppl. 1): S81–S85.
2. Messerli H, Schmeider RE. Blood pressure measurement in the elderly. In: O'Brien E, O'Malley K, editors, Blood Pressure measurement. Birkenhager WH, Reid JL, series editors, Handbook of Hypertension. Amsterdam: Elsevier 1991: 148–54.
3. Kannel WB, Brand FN. Cardiovascular risk factors in the elderly. In: Andreas R, Bierman EG, Hazzard WR, editors, Principles of geriatric medicine. New York: McGraw-Hill 1985; 104–19.
4. Amery A, Hansson L, Andren L, Gudbrandsson T, Sivertsson R, Svensson A. Hypertension in the elderly. Acta Med Scand 1981; **210**: 221–9.
5. Amery A, Birkenhager WH, Brixko P et al. Efficacy of antihypertensive drug treatment according to age, sex, blood pressure and previous cardiovascular disease in patients over the age of 60. Lancet 1986; **2**: 589–92.
6. Furberg CD, Black DM. The systolic hypertension in the elderly pilot program: Methodological issues. Eur Heart J 1988; **9**: 233–7.
7. Torriani S, Waeber B, Petrillo A et al. Ambulatory blood pressure monitoring in the elderly hypertensive patient. J Hypertens 1988: **6** (Suppl. 1): S25–S27.
8. The Systolic Hypertension in the Elderly Program Cooperative Research Group. Implications of the Systolic Hypertension in the Elderly Program. Hypertension 1993; **21**: 335–43.
9. Staessen J, Amery A, Birkenhager W et al. Syst-Eur: A multicentre trial for the treatment of isolated systolic hypertension in the Elderly. First interim report. J Cardiovasc Pharmacol 1992; **9**: 120–5.
10. Pickering TG, James GD, Boddie C, Harshfield GA, Blank S, Laragh JH. How common is white coat hypertension? JAMA 1988; **259**: 225–8.
11. Lerman CE, Brody DS, Hui T, Lazaro C, Smith DG, Blum MJ. The whitecoat hypertension response: Prevalence and predictors. J Gen Intern Med 1989; **4**: 225–31.
12. Ruddy MC, Bialy GB, Malka ES, Lacy CR, Kostis JB. The relationship of plasma renin activity to clinic and ambulatory blood pressure in elderly people with isolated systolic hypertension. J Hypertens 1988; **6** (Suppl. 4): S412–S415.
13. Silagy CA, McNeil JJ, McGrath BP. Isolated systolic hypertension: Does it really exist on ambulatory blood pressure monitoring? Clin & Exper Pharmacol & Physiol 1990; **17**: 203–6.
14. Cox JP, Atkins N, O'Malley K, O'Brien E. Does isolated systolic hypertension exist on ambulatory blood pressure measurement? J Hypertens 1991; **9** (Suppl. 6): S100–S101.
15. Shimada K, Ogura H, Kawamoto A, Matsubayashi K, Ishida H, Ozawa T. Noninvasive ambulatory blood pressure monitoring during clinic visit in elderly hypertensive patients. Clin & Exper Hyper Theory and Practice 1990; **A12**: 15–70.
16. O'Brien E, Sheridan J, O'Malley K. Dippers and non-dippers. Lancet 1988; **2**: 397.
17. Pickering TG. The clinical significance of diurnal blood pressure variations; dippers and non-dippers. Circulation 1990; **19**: 93–101.
18. O'Brien E, O'Malley K. The relationship of 24-hour ambulatory blood pressure measurement to target organ damage. Therapeutic Research 1993; **14**: 84–91.
19. O'Brien E, Atkins N, O'Malley K. Defining normal ambulatory blood pressure. Am J Hypertens 1993; **6**: 201S–206S.
20. Waeber B, Niederberger M, Nussberger J, Brunner H. Ambulatory blood pressure monitoring in children, adolescents and elderly people. J Hypertens 1991; **9** (Suppl. 8): S72–S74.
21. Floras JS. Antihypertensive treatment, myocardial infarction and nocturnal ischaemia. Lancet 1988; **2**: 944–6.
22. Stanton A, O'Brien E. Noninvasive 24-hour ambulatory blood pressure monitoring: current status. Postgrad med J 1993; **69**: 255–67.

23. Imholz BPM, Dambrink JHA, Karemaker JM, Wieling W. Orthostatic circulatory control in the elderly evaluated by non-invasive continuous blood pressure measurement. Clin Sci 1990; **79**: 73–9.
24. Rodstein M, Zeman FD. Postural blood pressure changes in the elderly. J Chronic Dis 1957; **6**: 581–8.
25. Zachariah PK, Krier J, Schwartz GL. Orthostatic hypotension and ambulatory blood pressure monitoring. J Hypertens 1991; **9** (Suppl. 8): S78–S80.
26. Lipsitz LA, Nyquist RP, Wei JY, Rowe JW. Postprandial reduction in blood pressure in the elderly. N Eng J Med 1983; **309**: 81–3.
27. Petrie JC, O'Brien E, Littler WA, de Swiet M. Recommendations on blood pressure measurement. Br Med J 1986; **293**: 611–5.
28. O'Brien E, Atkins N, O'Malley K. Selecting the correct bladder according to the distribution of arm circumference in the population. J Hypertens 1993; **11**: 449–50.
29. Staessen J, Amery A, Clement D et al. Twenty-four hour blood pressure monitoring in the Syst-Eur trial. Aging Clin Exp Res 1992; **4**: 85–91.
30. Silagy CA, McNeil JJ, Farish S, McGrath BP. Comparison of repeated measurement of ambulatory and clinic blood pressure readings in isolated systolic hypertension. Clin & Exper Hypertension 1993; **15**: 895–909.
31. Pickering TG, Devereux RB. Ambulatory monitoring of blood pressure as a predictor of cardiovascular risk. Am Heart J 1987; **114**: 925–8.
32. Cox J, Amery A, Clement D et al. Relationship between blood pressure measured in the clinic and by ambulatory monitoring and left ventricular size as measured by electrocardiogram in elderly patients with isolated systolic hypertension. J Hypertens 1993; **11**: 269–76.
33. Cox J, O'Brien E, O'Malley K. Ambulatory blood pressure measurement in the elderly. J Hypertens 1991; **9** (Suppl. 3): S73–S77.
34. Spence JD, Sibbald WJ, Cape RD. Pseudohypertension in the elderly. Clin Sci Mol Med 1978; **55** (Suppl. 4): 399–402.
35. Messerli FH, Ventura HO, Amodeo C. Osler's manoeuver and pseudohypertension. N Engl J. Med 1985; **312**: 1548–51.
36. Osler W. Principles and practice of medicine. New York: Appleton-Century 1892.
37. Finnegan TP, Spence JD, Wong DG, Wells GA. Blood pressure measurement in the elderly: Correlation of arterial stiffness with differences between intra-arterial and cuff pressures. J Hypertens 1985; **3**: 231–5.
38. Prochazka AV, Martel R. Osler's manoeuver in outpatients veterans. J Clin Hypertens 1987; **3**: 554–8.
39. Cox JP, England R, Cox T et al. Do subjects with stiff arteries have high blood pressure? J Hypertens 1989; **7** (Suppl. 6): 82–3.
40. O'Callaghan W, Fitzgerald D, O'Malley K, O'Brien E. Accuracy of indirect blood pressure measurement in the elderly. Br Med J 1983; **286**: 1545–6.
41. O'Brien E, O'Malley K. Clinical blood pressure measurement. In: Robertson JIS, editor. Clinical Hypertension. Birkenhager W, Reid JL, series editors, Handbook of Hypertension. Volume 15. Amsterdam: Elsevier 1992: 14–50.
42. O'Brien E, O'Malley K, Cox J, Stanton A. Ambulatory blood pressure monitoring in the evaluation of drug efficacy. Am Heart J 1991; **121**: 999–1006.
43. Wittenberg C, Zabludowski JR, Rosenfeld JB. Overdiagnosis of hypertension in the elderly. J Human Hypertens 1992; **6**: 349–51.
44. O'Brien E, Mee F, Atkins N, O'Malley K. Technical aspects of ambulatory blood pressure monitoring devices in the elderly. Cardiology in the Elderly. Cardiology in the Elderly 1993; **1**: 464–9.
45. O'Brien E, Petrie J, Littler WA et al. The British Hypertension Society Protocol for the evaluation of blood pressure measuring devices. J Hypertens 1993; **11** (Suppl. 2): S43–S63.
46. Miller ST, Elam JT, Graney MJ, Applegate B. Discrepancies in recording systolic blood pressure of elderly persons by ambulatory blood pressure monitor. Am J Hypertens 1992; **5**: 16–21.
47. O'Brien E, Atkins N, Mee F, O'Malley K. Comparative accuracy of six ambulatory devices according to blood pressure levels. J Hypertens 1993; **11**: 672–5.

3. Efficacy and tolerability of different antihypertensive agents with respect to age

GASTONE LEONETTI and CESARE CUSPIDI

Introduction

Hypertension in the elderly has been one of the most controversial aspects of cardiovascular disease during this century and only recently have enough clinical data been collected in order to justify the pharmacological and/or non-pharmacological reduction of elevated blood pressure values in people older than 60–65 years.

Hypertension in the elderly is a clinically relevant and socially important problem, since the duration of life has increased exponentially during the last century and the prevalence of elevated blood pressure in the elderly is higher than in young and adult persons [1]. In spite of that, the problem of hypertension in the elderly has become almost forgotten by doctors, and many explanations have been proposed to justify the non-approach of this hemodynamic alteration (Table 1). Indeed, the first epidemiological trials on the relationship between blood pressure and fatal and non-fatal cardiovascular events were devoted to young and adult people and therefore our knowledge about this relationship in the elderly is limited. On the other hand, great concern has been expressed about the possibility of reducing blood flow to such vital organs as the heart, the brain, the kidney, etc., in the elderly, while reducing systemic blood pressure, due to the characteristics of the hemodynamic profile and baroreflex function in the elderly. Concern has also been voiced about the possibility of an abnormal response of blood pressure to antihypertensive drugs, either as a greater or a reduced fall, and the chance of a higher incidence or greater severity of side effects. In spite of all this, the main explanation concerning the non-approach of hypertension in the elderly was that age did and does remain the most powerful predictor of mortality in the elderly.

Other perplexities about hypertension in the elderly are listed in Table 2. Elderly hypertensives can be considered to be special people in that their

27

Gastone Leonetti and Cesare Cuspidi (eds), Hypertension in the Elderly, 27–50
© 1994 *Kluwer Academic Publishers. Printed in the Netherlands*

Table 1. Hypertension in the elder!y

1. Limited experience as a risk factor.
2. Concern about reducing blood flow to vital organs.
3. Age is the most powerful predictor of mortality.

Table 2. Elderly hypertensives: some perplexities

1. Survivors: a) many years to "track" to hypertensive levels.
             b) resistant to blood pressure elevation.
2. Frequent secondary forms of hypertension (renal artery stenosis).
3. Diastolic blood pressure relatively low.
4. Different response to antihypertensive agents.
5. More prone to side-effects.

blood pressure elevation has been more gradual and only at an advanced age did they show abnormal blood pressure levels. On the other hand, elderly hypertensives can be considered also as hypertensive patients who have survived the ravages of elevated blood pressure and are therefore special people. Furthermore, the appearance of hypertension in the elderly is frequently a secondary form of blood pressure elevation and among these, renovascular hypertension is the most frequent form. Due to the age-dependent changes of large arteries, responsible for reduced compliance, the diastolic blood pressure levels are frequently normal and even low in old people and, therefore, isolated systolic or predominantly systolic hypertension are hemodyamic patterns more commonly found in the elderly.

However, all these concerns and perplexities have been overridden by the prospective epidemiological studies which have shown that: 1) hypertension is an important risk factor for fatal and non-fatal cardiovascular events in the elderly, and 2) the pharmacological reduction of elevated blood pressure significantly lowers the incidence of cardiovascular events, as shown by the meta-analysis of Staessen of the epidemiological studies performed before 1985 and, more recently, in the SHEP, STOP-Hypertension and MRC trials (see the corresponding chapters 6 and 7 in this book).

In this chapter, we will deal with two pragmatic and clinically relevant questions about antihypertensive treatment that were of great concern until a few years ago: 1) Is there a relationship between the antihypertensive efficacy and the age of the patients? and 2) Is the incidence and/or severity of side effects related to the age of the patients? In order to give an answer to each of these questions, we will separately review the major antihypertensive agents, which are diuretics, beta-blockers, inhibitors of angiotensin-converting enzyme (ACEI), calcium-antagonists, ketanserin for its supposed particular efficacy in the elderly, and, to a minor extent, the inhibitors of postsynaptic alpha 1-receptors.

Although Ferrari dealt with the changes of the cardiovascular system with age in Chapter 1 of this book, we think it could be worthwhile to summarize the basic alteration of blood pressure elevation in the elderly. Essential hypertension in the elderly (when compared to the young) is characterized by a rise in total and renal vascular resistances, a greater left ventricular mass, a reduced cardiac output and a low intravascular volume [2], while total exchangeable sodium is similar or only slightly elevated [3] and, finally, plasma noradrenaline concentration is increased and plasma renin activity decreased [4, 5].

Diuretics

Although diuretic drugs have been available since the 1920s, it was not until chlorothiazide was introduced in the late 1950s that they were used in the routine treatment of hypertension. Subsequently, they have been the cornerstone of antihypertensive drug therapy for many years and remain so in many countries.

The literature on diuretics in hypertension is abundant, but relatively little attention has been devoted to age-related responsiveness.

The major hemodynamic effect of thiazide diuretics in elderly hypertensives is a decrease in total peripheral resistances [6] and a little overall effect on cardiac output or plasma volume [7, 8], although a decrease in cardiac output has been found in some patients [9]. Blood pressure reduction, as with other antihypertensive agents, is related to pretreatment levels of blood pressure [7], while there is only a slight increase in the antihypertensive efficacy by using high as opposed to low doses of diuretics [7].

Antihypertensive efficacy of diuretics in the elderly

The antihypertensive efficacy of diuretics in the elderly has been reported in uncontrolled studies, in placebo-controlled studies and as a function of the age of the patients. While studies of the first and second designs are relatively frequent, studies concerning the effect of aging on the response to diuretics are scanty.

In uncontrolled studies [6, 10–13] in elderly patients with systo-diastolic or isolated systolic hypertension, diuretics significantly lowered elevated blood pressure values. Blood pressure reduction was already present after 4 to 8 weeks of treatment and remained constant thereafter.

In three placebo-controlled studies [14–16], the Systolic Hypertension Study in the Elderly (SHEP), the European Working Party in the Elderly Hypertensives (EWPHE) and the Medical Research Council study (MRC), the blood pressure reduction in actively treated elderly hypertensives was significantly higher than in the placebo control group. Furthermore, diuretics have been compared with other antihypertensive agents, especially beta-

Table 3. Incidence of total mortality and cardiovascular events in active and placebo treated groups in two age-different population: MRC 1985 (age 35–64 years) and MRC 1992 (age 65–74 years)

	MRC 1985				MRC 1992			
	Active	Placebo	Diff	p	Active	Placebo	Diff	p
Total cardiovasc. events	6.7%	8.25	−19%	<0.005	21.0%	25.2%	−17%	0.03
Ictus	1.4%	2.6%	−45%	<0.001	8.1%	10.8%	−25%	0.04
Coronary events	5.2%	5.4%		ns	10.3%	12.7%		ns
Total mortality	5.8%	5.9%		ns	23.9%	24.9%		ns

blockers, but on the whole, there was no significant difference in the blood pressure reduction among them [17, 18].

Finally, for what concerns the influence of age on blood pressure response to diuretics, results so far available were not uniform. Indeed, while Andersen [19], Schersten [20] and Rowland [21] found a greater blood pressure reduction in elderly than in younger hypertensives, other authors [11,22,23] found no relationship of blood pressure reduction with the age of the patients. However, it must be underlined that in some studies, the pre-treatment blood pressure was more elevated in the elderly, while in others the blood pressure values before therapy were not reported. Therefore, although some studies suggest that the hypotensive response to diuretics is greater in older patients, the reported differences appear to be minor and contrary data can be quoted.

On the other hand, studies that have used diuretic-based antihypertensive therapy have demonstrated a trend or a significant reduction in cardiovascular morbidity and mortality in elderly patients. A recent study by the MRC into elderly hypertensives (65–74 years) allowed a comparison of results with those obtained by the same organization with an equal antihypertensive approach in younger patients (35–64 years). According to these results, a reduction in cardiovascular events was very similar in the two groups (Table 3). However, in contrast with these encouraging results for the use of diuretics in elderly hypertensives, there is Morgan's report which found a doubling of incidences of mortality in patients treated with diuretics, when compared with patients treated with other antihypertensive agents [24].

Side-effects of diuretics in the elderly

As already reported in the introduction, there was, and in part still is, a concern that the incidence and/or severity of subjective and laboratory side effects in the elderly could be greater than in young and adult subjects. In spite of that, the evidence for this concern with diuretics is tenuous and objective information is sparse.

As in young patients, thiazide therapy in elderly hypertensives induces a fall in plasma or serum potassium, and an increase in urea, glucose and uric acid [6, 10, 25–27].

Hypokalemia is considered to be one of the most dangerous and at the same time, frequent biochemical side effects of thiazide diuretics, especially the still unsettled relationship with arrhythmias. In two studies [28, 29], no relationship was found between a patient's age and a tendency towards hypokalemia. The reduction in serum potassium was found to be unchanged after the first month of chlorthalidone therapy in the SHEP study [26], while in the MRC trial [30], the reduction in serum potassium was found to be progressive.

Short-acting thiazides or loop-diuretics are considered to be associated with a lower incidence of hypokalemia than longer-acting thiazides or chlor-'halidone [31], although this does not appear to have been studied specifically in the elderly.

In the EWPHE study [32, 33], where patients were treated with the association of hydrochlorothiazide and triamterene as the first step, glucose levels increased progressively in relation to the fall in potassium and were stable after one year of therapy. At the same time, there was a rise in uric acid concomitant with an increase in serum creatinine.

Hyponatremia is a well-known pharmacodynamic complication of diuretic treatment and it has been found frequently in the elderly [34, 36]. Thiazides, rather than loop diuretics, are usually implicated and the thiazide-potassium-sparing diuretic combination seems to be more prone to induce hyponatremia. Although death or neurologic damage can result in some patients, the prevalence of clinically relevant hyponatremia is considered to be very low: indeed, plasma sodium levels were not recorded in some studies, such as the SHEP [26] and MRC [16] studies, or only small and insignificant changes were reported, as in the EWPHE study. Finally, no significant changes in plasma lipid levels during diuretic treatment were found in the elderly patients in the SHEP study [26] and in the small VARDEN study [8], although in post-menopausal women given a high dose of chlorthalidone (100 mg/die for 6 weeks), a rise in atherogenic lipoproteins was found in contrast to pre-menopausal women [37–40].

Anecdotal reports of impaired cerebral function have been reported during antihypertensive treatment in elderly hypertensives and this raises the question of what effect diuretics have on cerebral blood flow. Traub [10] found no change in cerebral gray matter blood flow or cerebrovascular resistances during hydrochlorothiazide therapy in a small group of elderly hypertensives, further information is necessary. However, the report by the Hypertension-Stroke Cooperative group [41] of a lower incidence of stroke recurrence in diuretic-treated patients than those treated with other agents, is very encouraging.

Conclusion

Diuretics appear as the drug of first choice for the treatment of arterial hypertension in the elderly, as suggested by the MRC trial in the elderly, the EWPHE study, the STOP-hypertension trial and the SHEP study, where a reduction in cardiovascular events followed blood pressure reduction obtained with a diuretic-based treatment. Whereas these views are widely accepted, it is nonetheless surprising how little objective data exist regarding diuretics in the elderly. Indeed, neither pharmakinetic nor pharmacodynamic patterns have been extensively studied for most diuretics in the elderly versus young patients.

The advocated age-dependent efficacy of diuretics has not been clearly demonstrated and it is probably related to higher pre-treatment blood pressure levels, although their efficacy in the elderly has been clearly shown in different clinical trials.

The nature of biochemical side-effects is superimposable on that of younger patients and, except for hyponatremia, there is no substantial difference in the frequency and degree of their incidence.

Beta-blockers

Preliminary studies in essential hypertension have shown that between 40 and 60% of patients have an adequate control of blood pressure on monotherapy with a beta-blocker, and the hemodynamic changes associated with prolonged beta-blockade comprise a reduction in heart rate and cardiac output and a smaller decrease in systemic vascular resistances. Bearing in mind that aging, per se, is characterized by a reduction in heart rate and in cardiac output at rest and predominantly during exercise, one wonders if the pharmacodynamic profile of beta-blockers is different according to the age of the patients or, in other words, if there is an age-dependent antihypertensive efficacy and/or tolerability of beta-blockers.

In order to give a correct answer to this question, the protocol of the studies should be characterized as to the age and sex of the patients, excluding secondary forms of hypertension and the blood pressure should be measured as many times as possible. Furthermore, the trial should be randomized, prospective and placebo-controlled, and different age groups (at least 4) should be included.

Because no clinical study completely satisfies these criteria, Fitzgerald [42] has analyzed the literature from 3 different points of view: 1) a review of what experts have published on this subject; 2) an analysis of rational prescribing patterns of hypotensive agents in relation to age, and 3) a review of the clinical trials that meet some of the criteria described above.

Review opinion

Eighteen out of 30 reviews addressing the relationship between hypertension, age and its therapy (see Fitzgerald [42]) advised that in hypertensives with an age of between 50 and 55 years, diuretics and non-beta-blocking sympathetic inhibitors were preferable because beta-blockers showed less efficacy and increased incidence of side effects in comparison with other antihypertensive agents. However, it is surprising that 6 reviewers out of these 18 papers provided no evidence of their conclusions, 4 authors quoted the same paper by Buhler [43, 44] and Laragh quoted his own paper only [45]. Finally, 2 authors quoted the paper by Vestal, performed on normotensive subjects.

Contrary to this, the other 12 authors suggested that the antihypertensive efficacy of beta-blockers was not age-dependent, 3 authors reported no reference, and the other 9 reviewers provided 7 different references [46–52].

Prescribing pattern of physicians

According to two studies [53, 54], one in Northern Europe and the other in the United States, the first choice of antihypertensive agent in the elderly hypertensives was a diuretic, although this does not mean that beta-blockers are less effective. These results contrast with the Swedish National Board of Health which suggests that beta-blockers are equipotent to diuretics in hypotensive efficacy in patients aged 65 years or older.

Clinical trials of beta-blockers in elderly hypertensives

Although there are numerous trials concerning the effects of beta-blockers in the treatment of elderly hypertensives, none of them met the previously outlined criteria. In spite of that, 25 trials have been reviewed by Fitzgerald [42] and his conclusions were subdivided as follows.

Reduced effect of beta blockers with aging
There are 6 reports that suggest an inverse age-related hypotensive response to beta-blockers and Buhler was the first [43] to report such a result in a group of 137 patients with an age range from 20 to 69 years. Stumpe found a similar age-dependent diminution of the antihypertensive efficacy of nadolol in hypertensive patients [55]. Other studies [56–58] did confirm these results, although many protocol pitfalls lower the clinical significance of all these trials.

No reduction of the effects of beta-blockers with aging
The authors of 16 clinical trials on the antihypertensive efficacy of beta-blockers suggest that there is no difference in the blood pressure reduction caused by this class of agents according to the patient's age. However, from the analysis of the results, it appears that the comparison of the efficacy of a diuretic and a beta-blocker was the main interest of these studies. The Birkenhager conclusion that "age per se would be a fallacious gauge for predicting the effects of beta-blockers" [59] is probably more pragmatic and true.

Age-related tolerability of beta-blockers

Although the literature provides an overall impression that there is an age-related increase in adverse events associated with beta-blocker treatment, this impression is not substantiated by real data. Probably this impression is derived from two observations: 1) surveys among geriatric patients seem to show a general increase in the incidence of drug-related side-effects in the elderly, which, however, is not drug-related nor disease-specific [60], and 2) papers reporting the age-related changes in pharmacokinetic and pharmacodynamic effects, often contain extrapolations, suggesting that this alteration may cause a reduced acceptability of the drug by the patients. Furthermore, the incidence of side-effects found by the Boston Collaborative Study Group [61] was 5.6% in patients under 50 years and 12.4% in those over 60 years. However, in spite of the fact that the difference was not significant, as cautiously underlined by the authors, these data have been reported by many authors as a demonstration of a higher incidence of side-effects in the elderly than in younger subjects.

When comparing the nature of side-effects in the Boston Collaborative Group studies [61] and in the MRC trial [62], it appears that the side-effects were predominantly of a cardiac nature (bradycardia, hypotension, heart-block, cardiac failure) and, to a minor extent, related to the central nervous system in the first study, and almost exclusively related to the central nervous system in the second study, without any age-related relationship. Lewis [63], did not report an increased incidence of side-effects with age in a carefully evaluated group of 100 hypertensive patients treated with beta-blockers. In this study tired legs, cold digits and vivid dreams were the side-effects more significantly related to the agents.

In two historical comparisons [64, 65] between patients below and above 65 years, there was no difference in the side-effects pattern. Other studies with timolol [66] and acebutolol [67] and that of Coop [68] involving patients of 60–70 years old did not support the view of an age-related increase in side-effects.

Metabolic effect of beta-blockers

It is known that prolonged beta-blocker treatment is associated with alteration of the lipid profile, which is more evident when it is compared with that of the placebo-treated group. The lipoprotein alterations caused by beta-blockers are a reduction in HDL and an increase in LDL lipoproteins and triglyceride plasma concentration, which are less evident with beta-blockers with ISA. In spite of a general agreement on these beta-blocker-related changes, there are no studies where the effects of beta-blockers on lipoprotein are compared in patients of different ages.

Beta-blockers may have a modest effect on the carbohydrate metabolism, that is a slight increase in the plasma glucose level, which, however, is not clinically relevant in non-diabetic patients. However, as for lipid metabolism, the age-related effects of beta-blockers on the glucose metabolism have not been adequately studied.

Conclusion

Current practice in many countries suggests that beta-blockers are less used for the treatment of arterial hypertension in the elderly than diuretics and the newly available agents. While part of the reduced use of beta-blockers may be due to a higher incidence of concomitant disease which do contra-indicate the administration of beta-blockers (and it is well known that elderly frequently have different diseases), there are on the other side some papers that show a lower antihypertensive efficacy and a decreased tolerability of beta-blockers in elderly hypertensives.

The suggestion that the age-dependent reduction in renin secretion or in end-organ responsiveness to beta-receptor activation will reduce the hypotensive response to beta-blockers, remains speculative.

Angiotensin-converting enzyme inhibitors (ACE-inhibitors)

Among the different systems responsible for the control of blood pressure, three of them have been the target of antihypertensive therapy:

1. manipulation of sympathetic nervous system, both peripheral and central components;
2. sodium homeostasis;
3. the renin-angiotensin system.

Although one drug may have a quite specific site of action, its effects are widely spread and therefore the hypotensive effect is the result of an interaction on different homeostatic mechanisms.

However, with increasing age, the relative importance of the different homeostatic systems does change to any varying extent and also the pharmacokinetic of the drugs is differently influenced by aging. Therefore, antihypertensive agents should be investigated for their efficacy, tolerability and safety in people of different ages, because they may have different effects and the results obtained in one age group cannot always be extrapolated to other age groups.

For those drugs acting on the renin-angiotensin system, the antihypertensive efficacy should theoretically be reduced with aging because it is well known that plasma renin activity does reduce with aging, while renin-angiotensin system-independent agents should be more efficient in the elderly. However, as already stated, no drug lowers blood pressure by only one mechanism, and other mechanisms unrelated to one specific mechanism can equally lower the blood pressure. The angiotensin-converting enzyme causes inactivation of different vasodilating drugs and this mechanism may explain the blood pressure reduction caused by ACE-inhibitors in low-renin or anephric patients. Furthermore, it has been identified also a tissue renin-angiotensin system and the inhibition of this local system may play a role in the blood pressure homeostasis of this class of antihypertensive agents.

On the contrary, an increase in the hypotensive effect of ACE-inhibitors in sodium-deplete subjects, who have a marked activation of the renin-angiotensin system, should be borne in mind, as well as the accumulation of these agents in patients with reduced renal function, with a few exceptions for ACE-inhibitors with renal and hepatic routes of excretion [66].

The efficacy and tolerability of captopril and enalapril, as the most representative agents of this class of antihypertensive agents, will be separately analyzed and their results can be extrapolated to the new agents of this family.

Captopril

There is no sizable placebo-controlled study in the elderly addressing the question of age-dependent efficacy and tolerability of captopril and when such data do exist, they are related to small, often open or single-blind studies, where captopril is sometimes given alone and others in combination, usually with diuretics. Two post-marketing surveillance studies do contain enough information to assess the frequency of age-related side-effects of captopril.

The efficacy of captopril in the elderly has been evaluated by three authors with positive results. Corea [67], by comparing captopril and diuretic in the elderly over 65 years, found similar blood pressure reductions, while metabolic changes were present only in the diuretic-treated group. Creisson [68] has shown a normalization of blood pressure in 94% of elderly patients treated with the captopril-diuretic association, while in the placebo-group, normalization was found only in 37%. In this study, no biochemical or hematological abnormalities were found. Tuck [69], in a large group of elderly patients ($n = 99$), found a controlled blood pressure in 51% of patients treated with captopril 25 mg bid. In non-responders, the association of a lower dose of captopril with diuretic was more effective than doubling the captopril dose, although 5 withdrawals were observed only in the association-treated group. Similar results were reported in small groups of patients treated with captopril monotherapy or associated with diuretics.

Two post-marketing surveillance studies are available to evaluate the incidence of adverse events. In the US study [70] of 175 elderly patients treated with captopril monotherapy or in association with diuretics or other drugs, the most frequent adverse events were rush (6.3%) and taste abnormality (2.9%), while a reduction in renal function was the most common laboratory alteration, and four patients were withdrawn due to deterioration of renal function. In a more recently published English post-marketing surveillance study [71], over 13,000 patients with a mean age of 61 years were evaluated

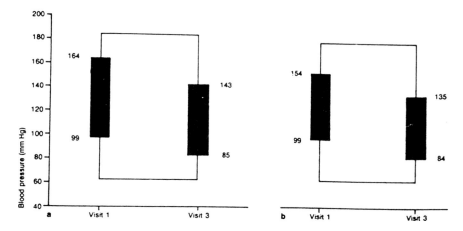

Figure 1. Mean blood pressure response to enalapril in: (a) elderly (>60 years of age, $n = 294$), and (b) younger patients (<60 years of age, $n = 672$) with uncomplicated mild to moderate hypertension (from ref. [131], with permission).

and, although it was not specifically addressed to the safety of captopril in the elderly, the authors commented that hypotension was present in 12 out of 6,057 persons under 60 years, and in 33 out of 7,238 above 60 years. Only 17 out of the total population (13,295 patients) were withdrawn due to renal impairment and 11 of them had had previous renal diseases.

Enalapril

Enalapril, as the most recent ACE-inhibitors which have become available after captopril, has been more extensively investigated for its efficacy and tolerability in elderly hypertensives (Figure 1). Reid [72–74] has investigated pharmacokinetic and pharmacodynamic profiles in young and elderly healthy volunteers during acute and chronic administration of enalapril, and found in elderly subjects a greater area under the curve (AUC) plasma concentration of the drug and a greater fall in blood pressure, although the degree of inhibition of the converting enzyme was similar in both groups. Therefore, the greater antihypertensive efficacy of enalapril in the elderly is due to the longer duration of the ACE-inhibition. The AUC of enalapril was inversely correlated with the patient's creatinine clearance.

In elderly hypertensives [75], enalapril caused an age-dependent blood pressure reduction when the blood pressure fall is expressed as an absolute systolic and diastolic lowering. However, if the blood pressure reduction is expressed as a percentage of the pre-treatment blood pressure levels, there is no more difference according to the age of the patients. As a consequence of the higher pre-treatment systolic and diastolic blood pressure (especially the former) in the elderly, the percentage of the patients who reached a target blood pressure (generally a diastolic below 90 mmHg) was lower in the elderly (55%) than in the younger group (73%). The most common side-effects were cough (3%), rush (0.5%), hypotension (0.3%) and angioneurotic edema (0.03%).

In conclusion, captopril and enalapril are efficacious antihypertensive agents in the elderly, while their relative efficacy compared to younger patients is more problematic, being in part dependent on the way of expressing the results. Post-marketing surveillance studies show that safety and tolerability are good, apart from the two major concerns; hypotension and renal impairment. Hypotension is more frequent in patients already on diuretic treatment, especially at high doses. Renal failure may be the consequence of bilateral renal stenosis more frequent in elderly hypertensives. Because most of the ACE-inhibitors are excreted through the kidney, the initial dose of ACE-inhibitors should be reduced in the elderly. Most of the concomitant diseases in elderly hypertensives do not contraindicate the use of ACE-inhibitors, but to the contrary, may be improved by ACE-inhibitor therapy.

Calcium antagonists

Among the different antihypertensive agents, the problem of an age-dependent efficacy and tolerability has been more extensively debated for calcium antagonists, although the reasons which have been proposed for this particular group, can be valid for many other agents.

As reported in another chapter of this book, the compliance of aorta and large arteries decreases with aging and this produces a disproportionate rise in the systolic blood pressure and impairs the sino-aortic baroreflex function, with reduced buffering of short-term blood pressure variations. Among humoral parameters, plasma renin activity has a trend to decrease, while plasma noradrenaline concentration is increased. However, due to the reduction in beta-adrenoreceptors, the beta-adrenoreceptors mediated functions are blunted with aging. In elderly, the blood volume and cardiac output are decreased and the renal function is impaired due to the reduction in glomerular filtration rate, renal plasma flow and concentrating capacity. Finally, the calcium content of arteries is augmented up to 100 times in the elderly when compared to infants. Therefore, aging is associated with pathophysiological adaptive changes in the cardiovascular regulation including reduced baroreflex sensitivity and beta-adrenoreceptor mediated cardiac and renal response.

As a consequence of these adaptive changes in older patients, there is a greater blood pressure fall for a given peripheral vasodilatation: indeed in the elderly, there is a minor activation of baroreflexes and a reduced rise in cardiac output, renin-release and water and sodium renal retention. Furthermore, if the vasodilating agents calcium antagonists are employed in the

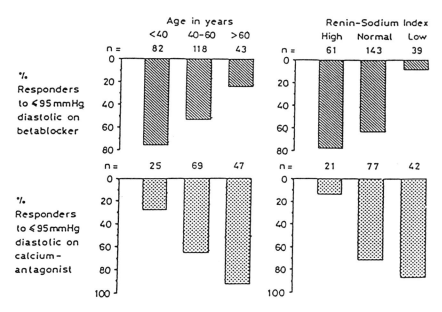

Figure 2. Percentages of blood pressure normalization (diastolic blood pressure <95 mmHg) during antihypertensive therapy with beta-blockers (upper panel) and with calcium antagonists (lower panel) as function of age or renin profile (from ref. [132], with permission).

elderly, their efficacy can be increased as a consequence of the increased calcium content of the smooth muscle cells.

Efficacy

Nicita Mauro in 1980 [76] was the first to report a beneficial antihypertensive effect of nifedipine in the elderly and similar results have been obtained by other groupls, using nifedipine [77–79], verapamil [80, 81] and other calcium antagonists, although no report has been published that this class of agents is ineffective in the elderly.

The problem, on the other hand, is more controversial when one considers the possibility of an age-dependent antihypertensive efficacy and tolerability. Indeed, the antihypertensive efficacy of calcium antagonists has been variously reported to increase with age [82–91], to decrease with age [92] or to be unrelated to age [78, 79, 93–99].

The suggestion of a positive correlation between calcium antagonists and age is essentially based on four studies of Buhler's group (2 with verapamil, 1 with nifedipine and 1 with nitrendipine) which were all non-randomized, single-blind and without a control group studies (Figure 2). All patients were treated in a sequential manner in order to reach a diastolic blood pressure below 95 mmHg or a certain dose of the agents. Two other studies with similar protocols confirmed the age-dependent antihypertensive efficacy of calcium antagonists, However, in spite of their assumption, Buhler has reported that according to a multiple linear regression analysis of his results, pretreatment blood pressure showed the strongest influence on blood pressure fall, followed by age and plasma renin activity [100].

According to a review by Chambers [101] there are only 3 well-designed studies, specifically aimed at comparing the antihypertensive efficacy of nicardipine [102], nifedipine [103] and nitrendipine [104] in young and elderly hypertensives. According to these studies, no difference in the magnitude of the blood pressure fall between the two groups was found. Although it is difficult to explain the differences between these three studies and Buhler's experience, it is possible that the different methodological approaches and analyses can explain part of the discrepancy.

Other studies found no correlation [105–109] and one reported a striking negative correlation [110].

However, a true correlation does exist between the fall in blood pressure and the degree of pre-treatment blood pressure which, however, is not specific of calcium antagonists, but is common for all approaches, placebo included. Because blood pressure rises with age a positive correlation can be obtained when the blood pressure fall is reported as an absolute blood pressure reduction, which, on the other hand is not found anymore when the fall is expressed as a percentage value.

In conclusion, calcium antagonists are effective antihypertensive agents in adult hypertensive patients of all ages, while there are no well-planned studies comparing the calcium antagonists' antihypertensive efficacy in young and adult patients that support the suggestion of a greater efficacy in the elderly. There is no doubt that calcium antagonists are generally equipotent to other antihypertensive agents. However, all these studies have been conducted predominantly in young and middle-aged patients and the few elderly patients investigated do not allow a conclusion to be reached.

The clearance of calcium antagonists in the elderly is generally reduced and the plasma half-life is augmented, but in spite of that, the effect of verapamil on atrio-ventricular conduction is not increased.

Adverse events of calcium antagonists in the elderly are similar to those of younger patients, although constipation by verapamil may be more troublesome in the elderly. Kuramoto [102] and Lopez [104] found a similar incidence of adverse effects in young and elderly patients, while Forette [111] found only one patient with adverse events in 35 patients aged 57–95 years. Different criteria for defining adverse effects may explain the different incidence found in various studies, but in spite of that, no trials showed an increased incidence of adverse events in the elderly.

Table 4. Baseline blood pressure levels and age-dependent degree of blood pressure reductions during Ketanserin and metoprolol or ketanserin and hydrochlorothiazide (from ref. [113])

Age	Ketanserin		Metoprolol		Ketanserin		HCT 2	
	Baseline	ΔDBP	Baseline	ΔDBP	Baseline	ΔDBP	Baseline	ΔDBP
<49y	107	−7.8	108	−11.7	108	−8.4	108	−10.8
50–59y	109	−11.7	107	−12.9	110	−11.4	105	−11.7
<60y	108	−14.7	108	−12.6	107	−15.3	106	−12.9

Ketanserin

Ketanserin is the only available agent for the treatment of arterial hypertension among the serotonin (S2) antagonists, which represent a new group of drugs, able to lower blood pressure in monotherapy as well as in a variety of combination regimens. Ketanserin has a complex mechanism of action. Indeed, it has been shown that ketanserin is not only a competitive antagonist of serotonin at central and vascular 5-hydroxytryptamine (5-Ht$_2$) receptors, but it also binds to α-1-adrenoceptors [112]. It is believed that its antihypertensive effect is the result of both central and peripheral actions [113, 114] and ketanserin has been shown to be equipotent to beta-blockers [115] and diuretics [116]. Furthermore, several studies have reported that ketanserin is more effective in reducing blood pressure in the elderly than in younger patients, during acute and chronic treatment.

Acute studies

The e.v. administration of 10 mg of ketanserin caused a significant fall in the systolic and diastolic blood pressure in a group of hypertensive patients with an age range from 25 to 90 years. While the systolic blood pressure was not related to the age of the patients, diastolic blood pressure was negatively correlated with it. In spite of that, there was an age-dependent reduction in the blood pressure of patients above 60 years of age, which was not correlated with baseline blood pressure. The reduction in blood pressure was due to a fall in total peripheral resistances [117].

Chronic studies

In the three subgroups of patients, randomized to ketanserin, hydrochlorothiazide and metoprolol by Rosendorff and Murray [118], the blood pressure reductions and the percentage of responders were greater in the elderly than in the younger during treatment with ketanserin and diuretics, while the opposite was found in the metoprolol treated group, but only the ketanserin change was statistically significant. All three groups had similar pre-treatment blood pressure values (Table 4).

In the Swiss ketanserin study [119], ketanserin alone or combined with atenolol or hydrochlorothiazide, was found to be more effective in lowering blood pressure in elderly (older than 60 years) than in younger patients. Other studies [115, 120, 121] confirm the age-dependent antihypertensive effect of ketanserin, unrelated to pre-treatment blood pressure levels.

Side-effects as dizziness, sonnolence and dry-mouth were those most frequently reported during ketanserin therapy and were more frequent in younger than in elderly patients.

Although there is no clear explanation for the greater efficacy of ketanserin in the elderly, some possible hypotheses have been proposed:

1) a more potent activation of the homeostatic mechanism in younger patients (but this should be valid for most antihypertensive agents);
2) a sodium retention in the younger patients, as suggested by a greater body weight rise in this group than in the elderly;
3) a selective enhancement of the blood pressure efficacy in the elderly due to some mechanisms not present or less active in the younger. This last possibility could be related to the more advanced degree of atherosclerosis in elderly which increases the vasoconstrictor action of serotonin and therefore the blood pressure reduction due to $5\text{-}Ht_2$ receptors blockade during ketanserin administration.

The slight differences in the pharmacokinetic profile of ketanserin between younger and elderly patients does not explain the age-dependent antihypertensive effect of this agent.

In conclusion, in spite of some negative studies, as that of Hedner [116], ketanserin does seem to have an age-dependent antihypertensive efficacy, although it is not known if this is a clinical advantage.

α-1-antagonists

Among the drugs able to antagonize α-1-adrenoceptors there are some with only this selective mode of action and others which have a mixed action: among the selective α-1-antagonists prazosin has been the most investigated while doxazosin has only recently become available.

Prazosin has a selective action on α-1-receptors and, therefore, does not interfere on the autoinhibition of noradrenaline release from adrenergic neurons and this can explain the limited rise in plasma renin activity, plasma noradrenaline and heart rate in spite of the peripheral vasodilatation and consequent blood pressure reduction [122, 123]. Prazosin has an effect on veins and arteries and therefore causes a fall in pre-load and afterload of the heart [124], while the incidence of central nervous system-related side-effects of prazosin is low and only at high doses [125]. Prazosin has been shown to lower the atherogenic lipoproteins and to rise the antiatherogenic ones [126], and recently it has been shown to correct the insulin resistance in hypertensive patients [127]. Prazosin has no clinically negative effect on many of the most common concomitant diseases in hypertensive patients.

Orthostatic hypotension is the most important side-effect of prazosin and is more frequent during initiation or increase of the therapy. Other factors, as size of the dose, fasting state, low sodium diet and previous beta-blocker therapy do exaggerate the first dose effect.

According to Stokes, prazosin is effective and well tolerated in elderly patients when administered as step 1 and eventually combined thereafter with diuretics, while it frequently causes persistent orthostatic symptoms when it is used as a step 3 drug [128, 129].

Meredith [130] has compared the antihypertensive efficacy of trimazosin and acebutolol in three groups of hypertensive patients (young, adult and elderly subjects) and, by expressing the blood pressure fall as a function of the plasma concentration of the drug, he found no age-dependent efficacy of the α-1-antagonist, while acebutolol was more effective in the younger group.

On the contrary, the impaired baroreflex sensitivity [131] and other factors, as neurological disease, venous pooling and reduced plasma volume, may contribute to the orthostatic hypotension caused by α-1-antagonists in the elderly, which is worsened by the concurrent beta-blocker administration.

In conclusion, the few available studies suggest that α-1-antagonists are as effective in the elderly as they are in younger groups. These agents have been shown to be neutral or to have a favorable impact on lipoproteins and insulin resistance, but, on the other hand, can cause orthostatic hypotension during initiation or increase of dose. The balance between the positive (blood pressure reduction and positive metabolic changes) and negative (orthostatic hypotension) effects should be evaluated for each patient before deciding. Recently, it has been suggested that there is a positive effect of α-1-antagonists in patients with prostatic hypertrophy.

General conclusion

Aging is associated with the alteration of various physiological functions and the vulnerability of older patients can be particularly exposed by all therapeutic agents, and among them, antihypertensive drugs. These and other reasons do not allow extrapolation to older people of what can be found in younger subjects either for pharmacokinetic and/or pharmacodynamic differences.

When treating elderly hypertensives, one wonders if the efficacy and tolerability of the antihypertensive agents are similar to those for younger patients and, according to the available medical literature, one is surprised to realize that very rarely have these problems been correctly approached in well-planned clinical trials.

Although diuretics are believed by many people to be more effective in the elderly, there is very little valid and objective information in relation to the age dependent efficacy of this class of antihypertensive drugs, while there is no doubt that they significantly lower blood pressure in elderly patients with systolic-diastolic or isolated systolic hypertension. Side effects in the elderly are similar to those found in younger patients, but hypokalemia, gout and diabetes mellitus are probably more frequent, as well as hyponatremia.

Beta-blockers form a class of antihypertensive agents which is differently employed in different countries. According to some authors, beta-blockers are less effective in the elderly than in the younger patients but, again, this has not been proved well. The same is true for the incidence and severity of side-effects, in spite of the fact that the antihypertensive efficacy of beta-blockers in the elderly is beyond any doubt, as are the chances of concomitant diseases which contraindicate their administration.

ACE-inhibitors do work in the elderly hypertensives, although there is no evidence that they work better. There are also no data of a higher incidence of side-effects in the elderly, although hypotension and renal function deterioration may be more frequent in the elderly.

The age-related antihypertensive efficacy of calcium-antagonists is one of the most debated problems in the field of hypertension therapy. Although there is no doubt about their ability to lower blood pressure, the data claiming their age-dependence may be criticized from a methodological point of view. On the other hand, it is true that many of the counterbalancing reactions, which can attenuate the antihypertensive effects of vasodilating drugs, are less valid in the elderly than in the younger people and this could allow more complete clinical evidence of the antihypertensive power of these agents in the elderly.

Finally, ketanserin is probably the only antihypertensive agent which has been correctly evaluated for its efficacy in patients with different ages, and the few available studies almost completely confirm a greater blood pressure reduction with this drug in the elderly than in the younger groups.

Apart from the lack of conclusive studies supporting an age-dependent efficacy of the more commonly used antihypertensive agents, we believe that other characteristics of the antihypertensive agents, as the contraindication or the indication, as a function of concomitant diseases, should be the guidelines for the selection of one drug or another. If the monotherapy with one agent does not allow us to reach the "therapeutic goal", it is always possible to reach it with an association with another drug and, therefore, the absolute blood pressure reduction is not a prerequisite for the selection of an antihypertensive agent.

References

1. Amery A, Hansson L, Andren L et al. Hypertension in the elderly. Acta Med Scand 1981; **210**: 221–5.

2. Messerli FH, Sundgaard-Riise K, Ventura HO, Dunn FG, Glade LB, Frohlich ED. Essential hypertension in the elderly: Haemodynamic, intravascular volume, plasma renin activity, and circulating catecholamine levels. Lancet 1983; **2**: 983–6.

3. Lever AF, Beretta-Piccoli AC, Brown JJ, Davies DL, Fraser R, Robertson JIS. Sodium and potassium in essential hypertension. Br Med J 1981; **283**: 463–7.

4. Schalekamp WH, Lebel M, Beevers DG, Fraser R, Koolsters G, Birkenhager WH. Body-fluid volume in low-renin hypertension. Lancet 1974; **2**: 310–1.

5. Padfield PL, Beevers DG, Brown JJ et al. Is low-renin hypertension a stage in the development of essential hypertension or a diagnostic entity? Lancet 1975; **1**: 548–50.

6. Varden S, Mookherjee S, Warner R, Smulyan H. Systolic hypertension in the elderly: Hemodynamic response to longterm thiazide diuretic therapy and its side effects. JAMA 1983, **250**: 2807–13.

7. Cranston WI, Juel-Jensen BE, Semmence AM, Handfield Jones RPC, Forbes JA, Mutch LMM. Effects of oral diuretics on raised arterial pressure. Lancet 1963; **20**: 966–70.

8. Vardan S, Dunsky MH, Hill NE et al. Effect of one year of thiazide therapy on plasma volume, renin, aldosterone, lipid and urinary metanephrines in systolic hypertension of elderly patients. Am J Med 1987; **60**: 388–90.

9. Van Brummelen P, Man in 't Veld A, Schalekamp MADH. Hemodynamic changes during long-term thiazide treatment of essential hypertension in responders and non-responders. Clin Pharmacol Ther 1980; **27**: 328–36.

10. Traub YM, Shapiro AP, Dujovny M, Nelson D. Cerebral blood flow changes with diuretic therapy in elderly subjects with systolic hypertension. Clin Exp Hypertens 1982; **A4**: 1193–201.

11. Niarchos AP, Weinstein DL, Laragh JH. Comparison of the effects of diuretic therapy and low sodium intake in isolated systolic hypertension. Am J Med 1984; **77**: 1061–8.

12. Plante GE, Dessurault D. Hypertension in elderly patients: A comparative study of indapamide and hydrochlorothiazide. In: Ogilvie RI, Safar M, editors. Indapamide and the current treatment of hypertension, London: John Libbey Eurotext 1986: 41–9.

13. Vardan S, Dunsky MH, Hill NE, Mookherjee S, Smulyan H, Warner RA. Systemic systolic hypertension in the elderly: correlation of hemodynamics, plasma volume, renin, aldosterone, urinary metanephrines and response to thiazide therapy. Am J Cardiol 1986; **58**: 1030–4.

14. Perry HM et al. Systolic hypertension in the elderly program, pilot study (SHEP-PS): Morbidity and mortality experience. J Hypertens 1986; **4** (Suppl. 6): S21–S23.

15. Amery A et al. European Working Party. Efficacy of antihypertensive drug treatment according to age, sex, blood pressure, and previous cardiovascular disease in patients over the age of 60. Lancet 1986; **2**: 589–92.

16. Medical Research Council trial of treatment of hypertension in older adults: principal results. Br Med J 1992; **304**: 405–12.

17. Forrest WA. The treatment of hypertension in older patients: a double-blind, between-patient study in previously treated patients comparing a diuretic, a beta-receptor antagonist, and their fixed combination. J In Med Res 1981; **9**: 490–4.

18. Wikstrand J, Westergren G, Berglund G et al. Antihypertensive treatment with metoprolol or hydrochlorothiazide in patients aged 60 to 75 years. JAMA 1986; **255**: 1304–10.

19. Andersen GS. Antihypertensive treatment in elderly patients in general practice (preliminary results). Acta Med Scand 1983; (Suppl. 676): 151–60.

20. Schersten B, Kuylenstierna J et al. Clinical and biochemical effects of spironolactone administered once daily in primary hypertension. Hypertension 1980; **2**: 672–9.

21. Rowlands DB, Glover DR, Young MA, Stallard TJ, Littler WA. Once daily indapamide in the treatment of the elderly and young hypertensive. Eur J Clin Pharmacol 1984; **27**: 397–405.

22. Rosendorff C, Murray GD. The International Study Group. Ketanserin versus metoprolol and hydrochlorothiazide in essential hypertension: only ketanserin's hypotensive effect is age-related. J Hypertens 1986; **4** (Suppl. 6): S109–S111.

23. Fagan TC, Conrad KA, Le SM, Simons JA. Hydrochlorothiazide: relationship of antihypertensive effect to age and physiological and biochemical effects. J Hypertens 1986; **4** (Suppl. 5): S513–S514.

24. Vardan S, Mookherjee S et al. Systolic hypertension in the elderly: Hemodynamic response to long-term thiazide diuretic therapy and its side effects. JAMA 1983; **250**: 2807–13.

25. Myers MG. Hydrochlorothiazide with or without amiloride for hypertension in the elderly. Arch Intern Med 1987; **147**: 1026–30.

26. Hulley SB, Furberg CD, Gurland B et al. Systolic hypertension in the elderly program (SHEP): Antihypertensive efficacy of chlorthalidone. Am J Cardiol 1985; **56**: 913–20.

27. Wikstrand J, Westergren G, Berglund G et al. Antihypertensive treatment with metoprolol or hydrochlorothiazide in patients aged 60 to 75 years. JAMA 1986; **255**: 1304–10.

28. Ramsay LE, Boyle P, Ramsay MH. Factors influencing serum potassium in treated hypertension. Q J Med 1977; **46**: 401–10.

29. Hollenberg NK, Bannon JA. The PACT study: Post-marketing surveillance in 47,465 patients treated with Maxzide (triamterene/hydrochlorothiazide). Am J Med 1986; **80** (Suppl. 4A): 30–6.

30. Medical Research Council Working Party on Mild to Moderate Hypertension. Ventricular extrasystoles during thiazide treatment: Substudy of MRC mild hypertension trial. Br Med J 1983; **287**: 1249–53.

31. Flamenbaum W. Diuretic use in the elderly: Potential for diuretic-induced hypokalemia. Am J Cardiol 1986; **57**: 38A–43A.

32. Amery A et al. European Working Party. Glucose intolerance during diuretic therapy. Lancet 1978; **1**: 681–3.

33. Amery A et al. European Working Party. Glucose intolerance during diuretic therapy in elderly hypertensive patients: A second report from the EWPHE. Postgrad Med J 1986; **62**: 919–24.

34. Kleinfeld M, Casimir M, Borras S. Hyponatremia as observed in a chronic disease facility. J Am Geriatr Soc 1979; **27**: 156–61.

35. Ashouri OS. Severe diuretic-induced hyponatremia in the elderly: A series of eight patients. Arch Intern Med 1986; **146**: 1355–7.

36. Abramow M, Cogan E. Clinical aspects and pathophysiology of diuretic-induced hyponatremia. Adv Nephrol 1984; **13**: 1–28.

37. Boehringer K, Weidmann P, Mordasini R, Bachmann C, Riesen W. Menopause-dependent plasma lipoprotein alterations in diuretic-treated women. Ann Intern Med 1982; **97**: 206–9.

38. Jackson G, Pierscianowski TA, Mahon W, Condon J. Inappropriate antihypertensive therapy in the elderly. Lancet 1976; **2**: 1317–8.

39. Wollner L, McCarthy ST, Soper NDW, Macy DJ. Failure of cerebral autoregulation as a cause of brain dysfunction in the elderly. Br Med J 1979; **1**: 1117–8.

40. Jansen PAF, Gribnau FWJ, Schulte BPM, Poels EFJ. Contribution of inappropriate treatment for hypertension to pathogenesis of stroke in the elderly. Br Med J 1986; **293**: 914–7.

41. Hypertension-Stroke Cooperative Study Group. Effect of antihypertensive treatment on stroke recurrence. JAMA 1974; **229**: 409–18.

42. Fitzgerald JD. Age-related effects of beta-blockers and hypertension. J Cardiovasc Pharmacol 1988; **12** (Suppl. 8): S83–S92.

43. Buhler FR, Burkart F, Lutold BE, Kung N, Marbert G, Pfisterer M. Anti-hypertensive beta-blocking action as related to renin and age: A pharmacologic tool to identify pathogenetic mechanism in essential hypertension. Am J Cardiol 1975; **36**: 653–68.

44. Buhler FR. Age and cardiovascular adaptation. Determinants of an anti-hypertensive treatment concept primarily based on beta-blockers and calcium entry blockers. Hypertension1983; (Suppl. III): 94–100.

45. Niarchos AP, Laragh JH. Therapeutic approach in essential hypertension of the elderly based on renin-sodium profile. Kidney Int 1979; **16**: 907 (Abstract).

46. Zanchetti A, Leonetti G. Hyperension in the elderly: Special considerations. In: Butler RN, Bearn AG, editors. The aging process: therapeutic implications. New York: Raven Press 1984: 175–89.

47. Hutchison S, Campbell LM. Beta-blockers and the elderly. J Clin Hosp Pharmac 1983; **8**: 191–9.

48. Chobanian AV. Treatment of the elderly hypertensive patient. Am J Med 1984; **77**(2b): 22–6.

49. MacDonald ET, MacDonald JB, editors. Drug treatment in the elderly. In: Drugs acting on the cardiovascular system. London: John Wiley 1982: 97–124.

50. Hutchinson B. Hypertension in the elderly. Can Family Physician 1981; **27**: 1579–86.

51. Opie OH. Beta blockade in the elderly. Lancet 1986; **1**: 733–4.

52. Amery A, Hansson L, Andren L, Gundbrandsson T, Sivertsson R, Svensson A. Hypertension in the elderly. Acta Med Scand 1981; **210**: 221–9.

53. Griffiths K, McDevitt DG, Andrew N et al. Therapeutic traditions in Northern Ireland, Norway, and Sweden: Hypertension. WHO Drug Utilisation Research Group (DURG). Eur J Clin Pharmacol 1986; **30**: 521–5.

54. Ray WA, Schaffner W, Oates JA. Therapeutic choice in the treatment of hypertension: Initial treatment of newly diagnosed hypertension and secular trends in the prescribing of anti-hypertensive medications for medical patients. Am J Med 1986; **81**: (Suppl. 6c) 9–16.

55. Stumpe KO, Overlack A. Diuretics, beta-blockers or both as treatment for essential hypertension. Br J Clin Pharmacol 1979; **7** (Suppl. 2): 189–97s.

56. Medical Research Council Working Party. MRC trial of mild hypertension: The principle results. Br Med J 1985; **291**: 97–104.

57. Bannon JA, Steward KA, DeLisser O, Schrogie JJ. Clinical experience with timolol malete monotherapy in hypertension. Arch Int Med 1986; **146**: 645–57.

58. Zacharias FJ. Long term clinical experience with atenolol. In: Cruickshank J et al. Atenolol and renal function. (Royal Society of Medicine International Symposium Series). London: Academic Press Ltd 1983: 75–87.

59. Birkenhager WH, de Leeuw PW, Kho TL, Wester A, Van Dongen R, Falke HE. Selection of hypertensive patients for treatment with beta-blockers. In: Maurer W, Schoming A, Dietz R, Lichtlen Pr, editors. Beta blockade. Stuttgart: George Thieme Verlag 1978: 113–21.

60. Weedle P, Parish P. Pharmaceutical care of the elderly, III: Adverse drug reactions. Br J Pharm Pract 1985; **7**: 16–8.

61. Greenblatt DJ, Koch-Waser J. Adverse reaction to beta adrenergic receptors blocking drugs: A report from the Boston Collaborative Drug Surveillance Programme. Drugs 1974; **7**: 118–29.

62. Medical Research Council Working Party. MRC trial of mild hypertension: The principle results. Br Med J 1985; **291**: 97–104.

63. Lewis RU, Jackson PR, Ramsey LE. Quantification of side effects of beta adrenoceptor blockers using visual analogue scales. Br J Clin Pharmacol 1984; **18**: 325–30.

64. Wikstrand J, Westergren G, Berglund G et al. Anti-hypertensive treatment with metoprolol or hydrochlorothiazide in patients aged 60–75 years. JAMA 1986; **255**: 1304–10.

65. Wikstrand J, Berglund G. Antihypertensive treatment with beta blockers in patients aged over 65. Br Med J 1982; **285**: 250–1.

66. Singhve SM, Duchin KL, Morrison A, Willard DA, Everett DW. Disposition of fosinopril sodium in healthy subjects. Br J Clin Pharmacol 1988; **25**: 9–15.

67. Corea L, Bentivoglio M, Verdecchia P, Provvidenza M. Converting enzyme inhibition v. diuretic therapy as first therapeutic approach to the elderly hypertensive patients. Curr Ther Res 1984; **36**: 347–51.

68. Cresson C, Baulac L, Lenfant B. Captopril/hydrochlorothiazide combination in elderly patients with mild to moderate hypertension. Postgrad Med J 1986; **62**: 139–41.

69. Tuck ML, Katz LA, Kirkendall WM, Koeppe PR, Rouff GE, Sapir DG. Low dose captopril in mild to moderate geriatric hypertension. J Am Geriatr Soc 1986; **34**: 693–6.

70. Jenkins AC, Knill JR, Dreslinkski GR. Captopril in the treatment of the elderly hypertensive patient. Arch Intern Med 1985; **145**: 2029–31.

71. Chalmers D, Dombey SL, Lawson DH. Post-marketing surveillance of captopril (for hypertension): A preliminary report. Br J Clin Pharmacol 1987; **24**: 343–50.

72. Hockings N, Ajayi AA, Reid JL. Age and the pharmacokinetics of angiotensin converting enzyme inhibitors enalapril and enalaprilat. Br J Clin Pharmacol 1986; **21**: 341–8.

73. Ajayi AA, Hockings N, Reid JL. Age and the pharmacodynamics of angiotensin converting enzyme inhibitors enalapril and enalaprilat. Br J Clin Pharmacol 1986; **21**: 349–87.

74. Lees KR, Reid JL. Age and the pharmacokinetics and pharmacodynamics of chronic enalapril treatment. Clin Pharmacol Ther 1987; **41**: 597–602.

75. Cooper WD, Sheldon D, Brown D, Kimber GR, Isitt V, Currie WJC. Post-marketing surveillance of enalapril experience in 11710 hypertensive patients in general practice. J R Coll Gen Pract 1987; **37**: 346–9.

76. Nicita Mauro V, Barbera N, Buemi M et al. Nifedipine in the treatment of arterial hypertension in the elderly: preliminary report. Geriatr Gerontol 1980; **28**: 357–64.

77. Ben-Eshay D, Leibel B, Stessman J. Calcium channel blockers in the management of hypertension in the elderly. Med 1986; **81** (Suppl. 6A): 30–4.

78. Kuramoto K, Yamada K, Miuashita H. Age and efficacy of calcium entry blocker in essential hypertension-double blind trial using nicardipine. Jpn J Geriatr 1986; **23**: 180–8.

79. Hiramatsu K, Yamagishi F, Kubota T, Yamada T. Acute effects of the calcium-antagonist, nifedipine, on blood pressure, pulse rate, and the renin–angiotensin–aldosterone system in patients with essential hypertension. Am Heart J 1982; **104**: 1346–50.

80. Abernethy DR, Schwartz JB, Todd EL, Lucki R, Snow E. Pharmacodynamics and disposition of racemic verapamil in elderly and very elderly hypertensive males. Clin Pharmacol Ther 1985 **37**: 177 (Abstract).

81. Abernethy DR, Schwartz JB, Todd EL, Lucki R, Snow E. Verapamil pharmacodynamics and disposition in young and elderly hypertensive patients. Ann Intern Med 1986; **105**: 329–36.

82. Buhler F, Hulthen UL, Kiowski W, Bolli P. Greater anti-hypertensive efficacy of the calcium channel inhibitor verapamil in older and low renin patients. Clin Sci 1982; **63**: 439–42s.

83. Hulthen UL, Bolli P, Buhler FR. Calcium influx blockers in the treatment of essential hypertension. Acta Med Scand 1984; (Suppl. 681): 101–8.

84. Buhler FR, Hulthen UL, Kiowski W, Muller FB, Bolli P. The place of the calcium antagonist verapamil in the antihypertensive therapy. J Cardiovasc Pharmacol 1982; **4** (Suppl. 3): S350–S357.

85. Erne P, Bolli P, Bertel O et al. Factors influencing the hypotensive effects of calcium antagonists. Hypertension 1983; **5** (Suppl. II): 97–102.

86. Muller FB, Bolli P, Erne P, Kiowski W, Buhler FR. Use of calcium antagonists as monotherapy in the management of hypertension. Am J Med 1984; **77** (Suppl. 2B): 11–5.

87. Kiowski W, Buhler FR, Fadayomi MO et al. Age, race, blood pressure and renin: Predictors for antihypertensive treatment with calcium antagonists. Am J Cardiol 1985; **56**: 81H–85H.

88. Buhler FR, Kiowski W. Calcium antagonists in hypertension. J Hypertens 1987; **5** (Suppl. 3): S3–S10.

89. Buhler FR, Hulthen L. Calcium channel blockers: A pathophysiologically based antihypertensive treatment concept for the future? Eur J Clin Invest 1982; **12**: 1–3.

90. Pedrinelli R, Fouad FM, Tarazi RC, Bravo EL, Textor SC. Nitrendipine, a calcium-entry blocker: Renal and humoral effects in human arterial hypertension. Arch Intern Med 1986; **146**: 62–5.

91. Fritschka E, Distler A, Gotzen R, Thiede H-M, Philipp T. Cross-over comparison of nitrendipine with propranolol in patients with essential hypertension. J Cardiovasc Pharmacol 1984; **6** (Suppl. 7): S1100–S4.

92. Ferrara LA, Fasano ML, Soro S. Age related antihypertensive effect of nitrendipine, a new calcium entry blocking agent. Eur J Clin Pharmacol 1985; **28**: 473–4.

93. Schulte KL, Meyer-Sabellek WA, Haertenberger A et al. Antihypertensive and metabolic effects of diltiazem and nifedipine. Hypertension 1986; **8**: 859–65.

94. Hallin L, Andren L, Hansson L. Controlled trial of nifedipine and bendroflumethiazide in hypertension. J Cardiovasc Pharmacol 1983; **5**: 1083–5.

95. Midtbo K, Hals O, Van der Meer J. Verapamil compared with nifedipine in the treatment of essential hypertension. J Cardiovasc Pharmacol 1982; **4** (Suppl. 3): S363–S8.

96. Singh BN, Rebanal P, Piontek M, Nademanee K. Calcium antagonists and beta-blockers in the control of mild moderate systemic hypertension, with particular reference to verapamil and propranolol. Am J Cardiol 1986; **57**: 99–105D.

97. Halperin AK, Gross KM, Rogers JF, Cubeddu LX. Verapamil and propranolol in essential hypertension. Clin Pharmacol Ther 1984; **36**: 750–7.

98. Ohman KP, Weiner L, Von Schenck H, Karlberg BE. Antihypertensive and metabolic effects of nifedipine and labetalol alone and in combination in primary hypertension. J Clin Pharmacol 1985; **29**: 149–54.

99. McMahon FG. Comparison of nitrendipine with propranolol and its use in combined cardiovascular therapy. Am J Cardiol 1986; **58**: 8–11D.

100. Kirkendall WM. Treatment of hypertension in the elderly. Am J Cardiol 1986; **57**: 63–68C.

101. Chalmers JP, Smith SA, Wing LMH. Hypertension in the elderly: The role of calcium antagonists. J Cardiovasc Pharmacol 1988; **12** (Suppl. 18): S147–S155.

102. Kuramoto K, Yamada K, Miuashita H. Age and efficacy of calcium entry blocker in essential hypertension — double blind trial using nicardipine. Jpn J Geriatr 1986; **23**: 180–8.

103. Hiramatsu K, Yamagishi F, Kubota T, Yamada T. Acute effects of the calcium antagonist, nifedipine, on blood pressure, pulse rate, and the renin–angiotensin–aldosterone system in patients with essential hypertension. Am Heart J 1982; **104**: 1346–50.

104. Lopez LM, Mehta TC, Fagan PC, Deedwania PC, Birkett JP. Is antihypertensive therapy with calcium channel blockers more effective in the elderly than in younger subjects? Presented at the Annual Meeting of the American Society of Hypertension. New York: May 1987. (Abstract n. A94).

105. Schulte K-L, Meyer Sabellek WA, Haertenberger A et al. Antihypertensive and metabolic effects of diltiazem and nifedipine. Hypertension 1986; **8**: 859–65.

106. Hallin L, Andren L, Hansson L. Controlled trial of nifedipine and bendroflumethiazide in hypertension. J Cardiovasc Pharmacol 1983; **5**: 1083–5.

107. Midtbo K, Hals O, Van der Meer J. Verapamil compared with nifedipine in the treatment of essential hypertension. J Cardiovasc Pharmacol 1982; **4** (Suppl. 3): S363–S368.

108. Singh BN, Rebanal P, Piontek M, Nademanee K. Calcium antagonists and beta-blockers in the control of mild to moderate systemic hypertension, with particular reference to verapamil and propranolol. Am J Cardiol 1986; **57**: 99–105D.

109. McMahon FG. Comparison of nitrendipine with propranolol and its use in combined cardiovascular therapy. Am J Cardiol 1986; **58**: 8–11D.

110. Ferrara LA, Fasano ML, Soro S. Age related antihypertensive effect of nitrendipine, a new calcium entry blocking agent. Eur J Clin Pharmacol 1985; **28**: 473–4.

111. Forette F, Bellet M, Henry JF et al. Effect of nicardipine in elderly hypertensive patients. Br J Clin Pharmacol 1985; **20**: 125–9S.

112. Vanhoutte P, Amery A, Birkenhager W. Serotoninergic mechanisms in hypertension: Focus on the effects of ketanserin. Hypertension 1988; **11**: 111–33.

113. Phillips CA, Myelcharame EJ, Markus J K, Shaw J. Hypotensive action of ketanserin in dogs: involvement of a centrally mediated inhibition of sympathetic vascular tone. Eur J Pharmacol 1985; **111**: 319–27.

114. McCall RB, Schuette MR. Evidence for an alpha, receptor mediated central sympathoinhibitory action of ketanserin. J Pharmacol Exp Ther 1984; **228**: 704–10.

115. Sheps SG, Schurger A, Zachariah PK et al. Comparison of ketanserin and metoprolol in the treatment of hypertension. Arch Intern Med 1987; **147**: 291–6.
116. Hedner T, Persson B, Berglund G. A comparative and long term evaluation of ketanserin in the treatment of essential hypertension. J Cardiovasc Pharmacol 1985; **7** (Suppl. 7): S148–S153.
117. De Crée J, Houig M, De Ryck M, Symoens J. The acute antihypertensive effect of ketanserin increases with age. J Cardiovasc Pharmacol 1985; **7** (Suppl. 7): S126–S127.
118. Rosendorff C, Murray GD (for the International Study Group). Ketanserin versus metoprolol and hydrochlorothiazide in essential hypertension: Only ketanserin's effect is age-related. J Hypertens 1986; **4** (Suppl. 6): S109–S111.
119. Beretta-Piccoli C, Amstein R, Bertel O et al. Antihypertensive efficacy of ketanserin alone or in combination with a blocker or a diuretic: the Swiss Ketanserin Study. J Cardiovasc Pharmacol 1987; **10** (Suppl. 3): S107–S112.
120. Cameron HA, Waller PC, Ramsay LE. Ketanserin in essential hypertension: Use as monotherapy and in combination with a diuretic or β-adrenoceptor antagonist. Br J Clin Pharmacol 1987; **24**: 705–11.
121. Symons J. Personal communication.
122. Davey MJ, Massingham R. A review of the biological effects of prazosin, including recent pharmacological findings. Med Res Opin 1976/77; **4** (Suppl. 2): 47–60.
123. Graham MR, Stephenson WH, Pettinger WA. Pharmacological evidence for a functional role of the prejunctional α-adrenoceptor in noraderenergic neurotransmission in the conscious rat. Naunyn Aschmied Arch Pharmacol 1980; **311**: 129–38.
124. Awan NA, Miller RR, Maxwell K, Mason DT. Effects of prazosin on forearm resistance and capacitance vessels. Clin Pharmacol Ther 1977; **22**: 79–84.
125. Fuller RW, Snoddy HD, Perry KW. Effect of prazosin on norepinephrine concentration and turnover in rat brain and heart. Arch Int Pharmacodyn 1978; **231**: 30–6.
126. Leren P, Foss PO, Helgeland A et al. Effect of propranolol and prazosin on blood lipids. The Oslo Study. Lancet 1980; **2**: 4–6.
127. Lithell H, Pollare T, Berne C. Insulin sensitivity in newly detected hypertensive patients: Influence of captopril and other antihypertensive agents on insulin sensitivity and related biological problem. J Cardiovasc Pharmacol 1990; **15** (Suppl. 5): S46–S52.
128. Stokes GS, Marwood JF. Review of the use of α-adrenoceptor antagonists in hypertension. Meth Find Exp Clin Pharmacol 1984; **6**: 197–204.
129. Stokes GS. Age-related effects of antihypertensive therapy with alpha-blockers. J Cardiovasc Pharmacol 1988; **12** (Suppl. 8): S109–S115.
130. Meredith PA, Kelman AW, Scott PJW, Reid JL. Concentration-effect analysis and its application in age-related studies. Br J Clin Pharmacol 1987; **22**: 605P.
131. Gribbin B, Pickering TG, Sleight P, Peto R. Effect of age and high blood pressure on baroreflex sensitivity in man. Circ Res 1971; **29**: 424–31.
132. Medina-Ruiz A, Feliu JF. A cooperative study to evaluate the efficacy and safety of enalapril in Puerto Rico patients. Drugs 1990; **39** (Suppl. 2): 77–82.
133. Buhler FR, Burkart F, Lutold Be, Kung M, Marbet G, Pfiisterer M. Antihypertensive beta-blocking action as related to renin and age: A pharmacological tool to identify pathogenetic mechanisms in essential hypertension. Am J Cardiol 1975; **36**: 653–69.

4. Treatment of hypertension and concomitant disease in the elderly

ARIE T. J. LAVRIJSSEN and PETER W. DE LEEUW

Introduction

Aging not only is accompanied by a gradual rise in blood pressure but also by an increasing incidence of other ailments. This poses an important problem on the treatment of hypertension in the elderly, because already two-thirds of patients above 65 years of age have a blood pressure exceeding 140/90 mmH [1]. Of them, some 25% have coexistent overt cardiovascular disease. In the elderly, hypertension is a very important risk factor for the development of cardiovascular complications, second only after diabetes mellitus, but still before hypercholesterolemia and smoking [2]. Clustering of risk factors increases the incidence of cardiovascular sequelae enormously and makes treatment directed at these risk factors mandatory. Hypertension therefore must be dealt with in the context of the entire cardiovascular risk profile. Table 1 shows the prevalence of risk factors as found in the Framingham Heart Study from 1970 to 1982. Except for these comorbid factors, hypertension may be accompanied by other diseases that have to be taken into account when instituting antihypertensive treatment (Table 2).

In general, the choice of an antihypertensive drug depends on several important factors such as efficacy of the drug, pharmacodynamic properties of the drug, profile of adverse effects, usefulness of the drug in cases of concomitant disease and concomitant medication, and costs of the drug. In this chapter, we will focus on the usefulness of antihypertensive drugs in patients with concomitant disease. For each of the disease states mentioned, we will discuss the specific properties of different classes of antihypertensive drugs currently in use, including diuretics, α-adrenergic antagonists, β-adrenergic antagonists, centrally acting drugs, vasodilators, calcium-entry blockers, angiotensin-converting enzyme inhibitors (ACE-inhibitors) and serotonin antagonists. Where necessary, we will discuss specific drugs separately.

Because hypertension in the elderly for many years was misjudged as a

51

Gastone Leonetti and Cesare Cuspidi (eds), Hypertension in the Elderly, 51–69
© 1994 *Kluwer Academic Publishers. Printed in the Netherlands*

Table 1. Prevalence of cardiovascular risk factors and disease in hypertension. (from: *Framingham Heart Study*, 1970–1982)

	Men	Women
Hypercholesterolemia	26.2%	51.8%
Low HDL cholesterol	14.3%	7.5%
Diabetes mellitus	20.1%	15.2%
Left venticular hypertrophy	10.1%	6.2%
Obesitas	22.1%	34.4%
Angina pectoris	12.2%	16.0%
Congestive heart failure	3.0%	4.9%
Stroke	9.5%	4.9%
Intermittent claudication	9.0%	6.2%
Total cardiovascular disease	31.4%	26.9%

Table 2. Frequently encountered diseases in the elderly hypertensive

Cardiovascular comorbidity	Metabolic comorbidity
left ventricular hypertrophy	diabetes mellitus
congestive heart failure	hyperlipidemia
coronary artery disease	gout
cardiac arrhythmias	
myocardial infarction	*Miscellaneous comorbidity*
cerebrovascular accident	chronic obstructive pulmonary disease
orthostatic hypotension	renal disease
peripheral vascular disease	benign prostatic hyperplasia
Raynaud's syndrome	mental/cognitive disorders
atherosclerosis	osteoporosis

minor health problem, most data on antihypertensive treatment, both with respect to effectiveness and with respect to adverse effects, have been obtained in studies on younger patients. Yet, it is possible to extrapolate many of these findings to the older population, at least as far as interference with concomitant disease is concerned.

Non-pharmacological antihypertensive treatment

As in younger patients, antihypertensive treatment in the elderly may include non-pharmacological interventions. However, as studies on non-pharmacological treatment have not yielded consistent results in the past, the usefulness of this approach must not be overestimated [3]. Both the data on the effectiveness of blood pressure control and those on the reduction of cardiovascular complications, have been disappointing. Nevertheless, in a subset of hypertensive patients, individual non-pharmacological interventions may be worthwhile to try and particularly in elderly patients non-pharmacological treatment can be useful [4].

Weight reduction has proven to be the most effective non-pharmacological antihypertensive intervention, especially when combined with modest physical exercise. Although data in this respect vary considerably, it is fair to state that reduction of body weight with 1 kg is associated with a drop in blood pressure, both systolic and diastolic, of 1 mmHg. However, physical exercise alone already has a place in the management of hypertension [5]. Such exercise should be dynamic, as static exercise is accompanied by a rise in total peripheral resistance and blood pressure.

The hypotensive effect of dietary sodium restriction varies greatly and cannot be predicted even though sodium sensitivity of blood pressure increases with age [6]. Restriction of alcohol intake can be effective as well; a limited intake is associated with lower blood pressures [7]. Other potentially useful non-pharmacological interventions may be the withdrawal of drugs that can raise blood pressure such as NSAIDs and sympathomimetic amines, and the cessation of smoking.

The major advantage of non-pharmacological treatment is the absence of any significant interference with most concomitant diseases or their treatment. On the contrary, non-pharmacological treatment often exerts a positive effect on concomitant diseases. For instance, weight reduction, physical exercise and limited use of alcoholic beverages may improve diabetic control, lipid metabolism and overall cardiovascular risk profile. Moreover, sodium restriction may especially be useful in case of concomitant congestive heart failure.

Pharmacological treatment

Cardiovascular comorbidity

Left ventricular hypertrophy
The prevalence of left ventricular hypertrophy (LVH) in the adult population as a whole is 15–20% and even 33% in patients over 70 years of age (Framingham study). From data of the same study LVH proved to be an independent risk factor for the development of cardiovascular events [8]. It predisposes to left ventricular dysfunction and cardiac arrhythmias. Regression of LVH can be accomplished with several antihypertensive agents: ACE-inhibitors, calcium-entry blockers, α_1-adrenergic antagonists, β-adrenergic antagonists, α-methyldopa and even diuretics have all been shown to cause reversal of hypertrophy. Recently, the same was found for a β-blocker with vasodilating properties [9]. Vasodilator drugs such as minoxidil and hydralazine do not cause regression of LVH. A meta-analysis of 109 studies, comprising 2357 patients, indicated that left ventricular mass (LVM) was reduced on average by 12% [10]. Whereas ACE-inhibitors, calcium-entry

blockers and β-adrenergic antagonists all decreased LVM through a reduction in left ventricular wall thickness, diuretics did so through a fall in left ventricular diameter. Reversal of LVH is believed to be mainly pressure related but, although not proven, some agent specific actions may play an additional role [11]. In this respect, the alleged superiority of ACE-inhibitors is attributed to their effect on arterial compliance and to the inhibition of the growth-stimulating effect of angiotensin II.

In hypertensive patients above 65 years of age regression of LVH, documented by echocardiography, can be shown already within three months following treatment with a calcium-entry blocker (nifedipine or nicardipine) or an ACE-inhibitor (captopril or enalapril) [12]. In the EWPHE-trial treatment of patients over 60 years of age with a diuretic with or without methyldopa for 4 years also appeared to diminish electrocardiographic signs of LVH [13].

Of paramount importance is the question whether the systolic function of the heart decreases pari passu with the regression of LVH, because the latter may be seen as an adaptive response of the heart to increased afterload. In 42 patients over 60 years of age, treated with verapamil or atenolol alone or in combination with chlorthalidone, systolic function remained intact after withdrawal of these drugs [14]. In contrast, the effect of regression of LVH on diastolic function of the heart is not yet clear.

Thus, most antihypertensive drugs cause regression of LVH, thereby decreasing the risk of cardiovascular complications. Regression of LVH during treatment does not impair cardiac performance.

Congestive heart failure
Congestive heart failure is not uncommon in the elderly hypertensive and may be attributed to underlying hypertensive and/or ischemic heart disease. Although most data on the effect of treatment of congestive heart failure on clinical outcome have been obtained in younger (normotensive) patients, there is no a priori reason why these findings should not be extrapolated to the older population. Diuretic therapy is the therapy of first choice in patients with congestive heart failure due to systolic dysfunction. The SHEP-study showed that the occurrence of left ventricular failure was significantly reduced during antihypertensive treatment with diuretics [15]. In case of obstructive abnormalities causing congestive symptoms, the judicious use of β-adrenergic antagonists or calcium-entry blockers may be indicated.

Certain vasodilators, and in particular, ACE-inhibitors have been shown to reduce signs and symptoms and to improve life expectancy in patients with congestive heart failure in WHO stage II–IV [16–19]. Yet, most of these patients were normotensive, not very old and already treated with diuretics. Nevertheless, one might expect ACE-inhibitors to be quite useful in elderly hypertensives with congestive heart failure. ACE-inhibitors reduce afterload, improve venous compliance, thereby reducing preload, enhance left ventricular diastolic function and decrease left ventricular hypertrophy.

Table 3. Cardiovascular effects of calcium-entry blockers

	Heart rate	Contractility	Conduction	Vascular resistance
Diltiazem	↓	↓	↓	↓
Diphenylalkylanines	↓	↓ ↓	↓ ↓	↓
Dihydropyridines	±	±	0	↓ ↓

↓ = decrease, ± = minimal effect, 0 = no effect.

Calcium-entry blockers reduce afterload and hence cardiac work by virtue of their arteriolar dilating properties. However, diphenylalkylanine calcium-entry blockers, and to a lesser extent diltiazem, have to be used with caution in patients with congestive heart failure because of their negative inotropic effects. Dihydropyridines, on the contrary, have little negative inotropic effect and may be used in these patients. The cardiovascular effects of the various calcium-entry blockers are shown in Table 3.

α_1-Adrenergic antagonists lower blood pressure by reducing tone in resistance and capacitance vessels, thereby unloading the heart. In chronic heart failure their use is restricted because of the development of tachyphylaxis. β-Adrenergic antagonists obviously are contraindicated in chronic heart failure. Yet, carvedilol, a β-blocking drug, exerting β_1-, β_2- as well as α-receptor antagonism, improves left ventricular work and well-being in patients with congestive heart failure. This improvement is positively correlated with baseline heart rate, suggesting primarily a beneficial effect of the reduction of heart rate leading to amelioration of diastolic function and coronary perfusion [20]. Finally, ketanserin, a drug with serotonin antagonistic and α_1-adrenoceptor antagonistic properties, reduces pre- and afterload without affecting cardiac contractility [21]. However, the drug cannot be used together with diuretics and its efficacy in chronic heart failure has yet to be proven.

Urapidil lowers peripheral resistance by means of blockade of vascular postsynaptic α_1-adrenergic receptors as well as by a central effect on 5-hydroxytryptamine receptors in the medulla oblongata. In congestive heart failure, a marked decrease in pulmonary vascular resistance is observed as well. However, whether this drug can play any role in chronic heart failure, is still elusive.

Coronary artery disease

In patients with coronary artery disease β-adrenergic antagonists are an excellent choice as antihypertensive drugs because of their cardioprotective and anti-anginal effects. They reduce heart rate and left ventricular stroke work, which in turn leads to a reduction in oxygen demand.

Calcium-entry blockers may improve coronary blood flow by dilating the coronary arterial system. Additional effects may be a slight reduction in heart rate (diphenylalkalines) and a reduction in platelet aggregation. Nifedipine seems to retard the angiographic progression of coronary artery disease although results have to be interpreted with caution [22].

Myocardial infarction
In patients suffering from myocardial infarction β-adrenergic antagonists remain the drugs of first choice because they improve post-infarction outcome significantly, mainly through a reduction in the incidence of cardiac arrhythmias. In case of severely compromised left ventricular performance they may however provoke clinically apparent heart failure. Under these circumstances treatment with diuretics, or better still ACE-inhibitors, is warranted. Diuretic-induced hypokalemia and hypomagnesemia should be avoided in view of the risk of arrhythmias. ACE-inhibitors have a beneficial effect on the left ventricle after myocardial infarction [23]. They attenuate myocyte necrosis and the reparative and reactive myocardial fibrosi [24]. Moreover, ACE-inhibitors decrease the incidence of serious cardiac arrhythmias in the post-myocardial infarction period [25].

In the past, vasodilating antihypertensive drugs have been used extensively in this context and they proved to be safe and effective with regard to the reduction of symptoms of dyspnea and fatigue, although they tend to increase heart rate. So far, calcium-entry blockers have not been unequivocally proven to improve survival after myocardial infarction. α_1-adrenergic antagonists and central acting drugs have no additional beneficial effect as do the drugs mentioned above.

The extent of blood pressure reduction to aim for is still a matter of debate. When blood pressure is lowered too far, coronary perfusion may become compromised, thereby imposing an increased risk for further coronary events. The existence of this phenomenon, known as the J-shaped curve relationship, is, however, controversial.

Cardiac arrhyhmias
Cardiac arrhythmias in elderly patients often are secondary to acute cardiac events such as myocardial infarction or to the use of diuretic drugs which may cause electrolyte disturbances, especially hyper- and hypokalemia and hypomagnesemia. Hyperkalemia may occur with potassium-sparing diuretic therapy in patients with a compromised renal function. Combination with ACE-inhibitors or NSAIDs under such circumstances may even provoke lethal arrhythmias. Hypokalemia may be dangerous in patients receiving digitalis and in patients who are already being treated with ketanserin [26]. In patients, suffering from brady-arrhythmias, sick-sinus syndrome and severe conduction disturbances (heart-block) β-adrenergic antagonists, verapamil, diltiazem and even centrally acting agents may provoke cardiovascular collapse and asystole as they are capable of decreasing the automaticity of sino-atrial and atrio-ventricular nodes and of the conduction pathways. In patients with high blood pressure and tachyarrhythmias, on the other hand, β-adrenergic antagonists may be useful in controlling these abnormalities and may

be considered as first choice. The most frequent tachyarrhythmia in the older hypertensive is atrial fibrillation. In case β-adrenergic antagonists are contraindicated, diphenylalkaline calcium-entry blockers may be of use.

Cerebrovascular accident
In the acute phase of a cerebrovascular accident severe increases in blood pressure may occur. In general, it is advisable not to treat high blood pressure in the acute phase [27], in part because blood pressure in most cases falls after the second day [28]. Treatment with nimodipine is beneficial because it improves neurological prognosis in particular despite the lack of an effect on the blood pressure level [29].

Orthostatic hypotension
The prevalence of orthostatic hypotension in normotensive and hypertensive independently living elderly subjects was reported to be 6–10% [30]. Surprisingly, the extent of the postural fall in blood pressure in this study was not related to the use of antihypertensive medication. Apart from an orthostatic fall in blood pressure a post-prandial blood pressure drop may also occur. Treatment of (supine) hypertension in patients with orthostatic hypotension can be extremely difficult. Control of orthostatic hypotension is essential because it may lead to collapse with all of the possible sequelae including ischemic cerebral damage, fractures, etc. In such cases hypovolemia and drugs interfering with adrenergic function should be avoided, if possible. Leg exercise and supportive stockings decrease venous pooling, thereby increasing venous return to the heart and improving cardiac output. A great number of venoconstrictor agents have been used in the past, albeit with little success. Supine hypertension even may be aggravated by these agents. So, the initial step must be the optimalisation of blood volume through dietary measures and in exceptional cases the administration of mineralocorticoids. The use of venodilators, sympatholytic agents and diuretics should be avoided at all times.

Peripheral vascular disease
In case of obstructive peripheral vascular disease β-adrenergic antagonists may further reduce blood flow in the extremities secondary to the fall in cardiac output.

In contrast, calcium-entry blockers are very useful in patients with peripheral vascular disease. The dihydropiridines are the most powerful vasodilators of these class of agents while diltiazem is the weakest.

Ketanserin is known for its vasodilating properties in patients with peripheral vascular disease. It improves symptoms in patients with intermittent claudication [31] and may therefore be regarded as a good choice in patients with high blood pressure and peripheral vascular disease. The results of the PACK-study, however, are disappointing [26]: no preventive effect of ketanserin on the incidence of thrombotic complications of vascular disease could be shown.

Raynaud's syndrome
In patients with Raynaud's syndrome β-adrenergic antagonists are not recommended. α-adrenergic antagonists cause peripheral vasodilation, thereby improving symptoms. Until now, calcium-entry blockers are the first choice under these circumstances.

Ketanserin promises to be a good alternative for the treatment of hypertension in patients with Raynaud's syndrome because of its vasodilating properties and its effects on platelet function. Yet, its usefulness has to be proven in clinical studies.

Atherosclerosis
In models of experimental atherosclerosis beneficial effects have been described for ACE-inhibitors, calcium-entry blockers, α-adrenergic antagonists and even β-adrenergic antagonists [32]. For instance, in animals fed a high-cholesterol diet, calcium-entry blockers inhibited the development of atherosclerotic lesions although the exact mechanism still is not known [33].

Studies investigating the effect of antihypertensive drugs on the development of atherosclerosis in humans are difficult to interpret because of changes in concurrent risk factors, different methods of evaluation and the inclusion of normotensive subjects, rather than hypertensive subjects. Slowing down of the atherosclerotic process in the coronary system has been shown for different types of calcium-entry blockers (nicardipine [34], nifedipine [35] and verapamil [36]). In the MIDAS-study the effects of isradipine and hydrochlorothiazide on the progression or regression of early carotid atherosclerosis are compared, but the final results are not yet available [37]. In the PACK-study a protective effect of ketanserin against cardiovascular complications in patients with claudication was suggested [26]. Although conclusive evidence that ketanserin retards the development of atherosclerotic lesions is lacking, studies in cholesterol-fed rabbits indicate that this drug may slow down lipid accumulation in arteriosclerotic lesions [38].

Metabolic comorbidity

Diabetes mellitus
Glucose intolerance may be seen in 15–18% of hypertensive subjects. Hypertension often is seen in the context of the so-called syndrome-X (insulin resistance, hyperinsulinemia, glucose intolerance, increased triglycerides and decreased HDL-cholesterol in combination with hypertension). The syndrome-X is found in up to 12% of the hypertensive population [39]. Management has to start with weight reduction, dietary manipulation (sodium restriction, reduced fat intake) and physical exercise. Antihypertensive treatment may on the one hand exacerbate the metabolic aspects of diabetes mellitus

(hyperglycaemia, lipid profile) but, on the other hand, favorably alter the course of diabetic nephropathy (proteinuria, glomerular filtration rate).

For years it has been known that thiazide diuretics may induce glucose-intolerance. In contrast, metabolic control in hypertensives with type II diabetes is not altered by nitrendipine [40] and nifedipine even seems to improve insulin resistance [41]. In addition, calcium-entry blockers may prevent progression of diabetic atherosclerotic disease by decreasing platelet aggregation [42], by altering lipid uptake and decreasing cell necrosis [33] and by inhibition of intimal cell proliferation [43]. Because of their β_2-receptor mediated effects on insulin and glucagon release, gluconeogenesis, glycogenolysis and adipose tissue lipolysis, β-adrenergic antagonists may induce variable alterations in glucose tolerance. The development or aggravation of insulin resistance, however, seems to be the most frequent mechanism seen with β-adrenergic antagonists [44, 45]. Although insulin sensitivity is improved by the α_1-adrenergic antagonist prazosin under experimental conditions, glycemic control did not change in clinical trials [46]. Of the ACE-inhibitors, captopril proved to decrease insulin resistance [47].

Several animal studies have demonstrated a decrease in proteinuria and improvement of glomerular filtration rate with the correction of systemic and intraglomerular hypertension. In these studies it was shown that ACE-inhibitors are more effective in this respect than calcium-entry blockers or a combination therapy consisting of vasodilators with diuretics [48, 49]. In clinical studies employing ACE-inhibitors, comparable results have been obtained, although separation of the effects of lowering systemic blood pressure from those of changing glomerular hemodynamics is difficult in humans [50]. In normotensive diabetics with micro-albuminuria captopril stabilized glomerular filtration rate and extent of albuminuria without any change in blood pressure [51]. The anti-proteinuric effect of ACE-inhibitors, therefore, is attributed to altered intraglomerular hemodynamics and possibly to effects on glomerular mesangial cells and the glomerular ultrafiltration coefficient [52].

The rate of decline in glomerular filtration rate in diabetic nephropathy is closely correlated to the level of blood pressure. Adequate antihypertensive treatment slows down the rate of progression of renal insufficiency and even after 10 years this beneficial effect still is apparent [53].

Evidence is accumulating that calcium-entry blockers may have the same beneficial effects with respect to the development and progression of diabetic nephropathy [54].

Hyperlipidemia
The effect of various antihypertensive drugs on the serum lipid profile is schematically depicted in Table 4. Adverse effects of antihypertensive treatment with diuretics on serum lipids are well known [55]. Although most types of diuretics have adverse effects on the serum lipid profile, thiazide diuretics are notorious for it. During the early months of treatment with

Table 4. Changes in lipid profile induced by various antihypertensive drugs

	Total cholesterol	LDL cholesterol	HDL cholesterol	Triglycerides
Diuretics	↑	↑	±	↑
Calcium-entry blockers	0	0	0 ↑	0
ACE-inhibitors	0	0	0	0
α-adrenergic antagonists	↓	0 ↓	↑	↓
β-adrenergic antagonists				
non-selective	↑ ↓	↑ ↓	↓	↑
β_1-selective	↑ ↓	↑ ↓	↓	↑
with PAA	0 ↓	0 ↓	0	0
dual	↓	↓	0 ↑	↓

PAA = partial agonistic activity, ↑ = increase, ↓ = decrease, ↑ ↓ = inconsistent reports, 0 = no effect, ± = minimal effect.

thiazide diuretics, serum cholesterol rises, albeit to a modest degree. However, serum cholesterol seems to decrease to pre-treatment levels thereafter [56]. In contrast to thiazide diuretics, indapamide is reported to be lipid neutral [45]. Whether these changes in lipid profile have clinical importance remains yet to be established.

The effects of β-adrenergic antagonists on lipid profiles depend on their pharmacological properties. Changes in lipids are due to an altered balance between β-adrenergic receptor mediated stimulation and α-adrenergic receptor mediated inhibition of lipoprotein lipase activity. Non-selective β-adrenergic antagonists decrease HDL-cholesterol and increase VLDL-cholesterol and triglycerides. They have no effect on total or LDL-cholesterol. β_1-adrenergic antagonists have similar, albeit weaker, effects. β-adrenergic antagonists with partial agonistic activity (PAA), on the other hand, are considered to be lipid neutral. β-adrenergic antagonists, with β_1-antagonistic, β_2-agonistic and vasodilating properties decrease total cholesterol, LDL-cholesterol and triglycerides. In addition they increase HDL-cholesterol [57]. Carvedilol, a drug with β-adrenergic and α_1-adrenergic blocking properties does not influence lipid profile [58]. As in the case of diuretic therapy, the clinical importance of such changes is not clear.

α-Adrenergic antagonists reduce triglycerides, total and LDL cholesterol and increase HDL-cholesterol [55, 59]. α-adrenergic antagonists may have a direct effect on LDL-receptor activity [60], or on cellular cholesterol levels [61]. The change in HDL-cholesterol is related mainly to a change in HDL_2 cholesterol.

Calcium-entry blockers have no adverse effects on lipid metabolism adversely. HDL-cholesterol increases without a change in the other lipids/lipoproteins during treatment with verapamil [62], diltiazem [63] or nifedipine [41].

ACE-inhibitors are lipid neutral and may even be beneficial [55, 64]. Abnormalities in lipid metabolism in non-insulin dependent diabetes mellitus are different from lipid abnormalities in non-diabetics. In the former most frequently an increase in serum triglycerides and a reduction in HDL-cholesterol is found, with lesser changes in total and LDL-cholesterol. Extrapolation of data from non-diabetic populations to diabetics, therefore, must be done with caution. Nevertheless, it is not unreasonable to presume that the effects of antihypertensive treatment on lipid metabolism will differ between these two populations.

Miscellaneous comorbidity

Non-diabetic renal disease
In the elderly, non-diabetic renal disease is not uncommon. About 6% of all hypertensive patients have renal dysfunction as defined by a serum creatinine above 135 µmol/l [65]. About 7% of the hypertensive population has dipstick proteinuria of at least 1+ and 20–30% even has significant microalbuminuria, i.e. > 15 µg/min.

Non-diabetic renal disease may be the consequence of long-standing hypertension but, conversely, it also may lead to hypertension. Deterioration of renal function is correlated, amongst others, to the height of blood pressure level and therefore it can be hypothesized that antihypertensive treatment diminishes the rate of deterioration. There are data to suggest that ACE-inhibitors are more effective in retarding the progression of renal failure than combination treatment consisting of β-adrenergic antagonists, vasodilators and diuretics [66, 67]. Antihypertensive treatment with calcium-entry blockers decreases the rate of progression of renal failure by as much as 50% [68, 54].

In the setting of chronic renal failure diuretics can be very useful because exchangeable sodium is often increased. However, diuretics tend to reduce renal blood flow and glomerular filtration rate by 10–15% [69]. This may lead to a significant increase in serum creatinine, especially in older (and diabetic) patients [70]. When glomerular filtration rate falls below 25–30 ml/min thiazide diuretics lose their efficacy and loop diuretics are needed.

Non-selective β-adrenergic antagonists also may impair renal hemodynamics [71] and cause a reduction in renal blood flow and glomerular filtration rate of 10–15% [69]. It is unlikely that the decrease in renal blood flow is the consequence only of a fall in cardiac output. Additional mechanisms, such as local intrarenal vasoconstriction, secondary to blockade of intrarenal β_2-receptors [72] may also play a role. Preservation of renal blood flow has been shown for the non-selective β-adrenergic antagonists tertatolol [73] and nadolol [74]. Data on the effect of β-adrenergic antagonists on proteinuria are conflicting. Yet, in several studies β-adrenergic antagonists reduced proteinuria [75, 76].

α-adrenergic antagonists, in general, do not have clinically important effects on renal hemodynamics or other aspects of renal function [77].

Combination of a β_1-adrenergic antagonist with an α_1-adrenergic antagonist (labetalol) likewise does not compromise renal hemodynamics [78]. Recently, β-adrenergic antagonists have been developed with vasodilating properties. Carvedilol, for instance, displays non-selective β-adrenergic blocking activity in combination with α_1-adrenergic blocking and possibly also calcium-entry blocking properties.

Although there is no uniform agreement, it has been suggested that calcium-entry blockers cause renal vasodilation in hypertensive patients, preferentially at the afferent arteriolar level, thereby increasing glomerular filtration rate and, above all, filtration fraction [79].

The effects of non-specific vasodilators on renal hemodynamics largely depend on their blood pressure lowering effect.

In patients with essential hypertension, ACE-inhibitors increase renal blood flow in spite of a reduction in renal perfusion pressure. Various ACE-inhibitors may induce disparate hemodynamic responses, probably related to pharmacokinetic and pharmacodynamic properties or as has been suggested also, they may induce different changes in the local intrarenal renin–angiotensin system [80]. ACE-inhibitors not only decrease proteinuria in normotensive and hypertensive diabetics, but also in hypertensive non-diabetics [81, 82]. Special attention has to be paid to the use of ACE-inhibitors in hypertensive patients with concomitant non-diabetic renal disease. When the existence of renal artery stenosis is suspected it is mandatory to exclude this condition as rapid deterioration of the renal function may ensue during ACE-inhibitor treatment. Although renal dysfunction usually is reversible after discontinuation of the ACE-inhibitor, renal insufficiency may persist when, for instance, renal arterial thrombosis has occurred [83]. In case of appreciable renal dysfunction, the use of ACE-inhibitors may lead to life-threatening hyperkalemia, especially when combined with potassium-sparing diuretics. So, monitoring of serum creatinine and serum potassium during ACE-inhibitor therapy is warranted.

Cognitive/mental dysfunction

As with increasing age cognitive function often declines, the prevalence of the combination of hypertension and cognitive dysfunction is fairly high. Both hypertension itself and antihypertensive drugs may influence cognitive function. Therefore, it is difficult to obtain firm and clearcut data on the evolution of the cognitive function during antihypertensive therapy. In addition, the ideal 'tools' to measure cognitive function have not yet been established. In 598 healthy community-resident subjects over 70 years of age, the cognitive function, as determined by Mini-Mental State Examination (MMSE), was highly correlated with blood pressure. The higher the blood pressure, the lower the score on the MMSE [84].

Diuretic therapy with hydrochlorothiazide has no adverse effect on the cognitive function [85]. As in younger hypertensive patients, treatment with captopril or nifedipine improved psychomotor performance in patients over 60 years of age within 1 week [86]. This improvement may be related to improvement of cerebral autoregulation. Psychomotor impairment for all has been described during the use of centrally acting antihypertensive drugs and β-adrenergic antagonists. Centrally acting drugs may depress central nervous system function causing depression, confusion or even pseudodementia. Central nervous system effects of β-adrenergic antagonists are inconsistent and do not correlate with lipophilicity [87]. Psychomotor dysfunction was not found in normotensive volunteers receiving an ACE-inhibitor (enalapril, captopril) or a calcium-entry blocker (nifedipine) [88–90].

A separate remark has to be made on the use of diuretics in patients receiving lithium therapy. Diuretics decrease tubular excretion of lithium, thereby increasing the risk of lithium intoxication. This combination should best be avoided.

Chronic obstructive pulmonary disease
In patients with a history of obstructive pulmonary symptoms β-adrenergic antagonists are contraindicated. Although some have advocated the use of β₁-adrenergic antagonists in patients with obstructive pulmonary disease, airway obstruction cannot always be avoided. ACE-inhibitors may produce an irritating dry cough but this is annoying rather than dangerous.

Gout
Diuretics decrease renal excretion of uric acid thereby causing hyperuricemia and increasing the incidence of clinical apparent gouty arthritis.

Nephrolithiasis
Thiazide diuretics reduce renal excretion of calcium and therefore are to be preferred in hypertensive patients with calcium-containing stones and in patients with hypercalciuria.

Migraine
Dihydropyridine calcium-entry blockers and non-specific vasodilators may provoke or aggravate attacks of migraine. They are best avoided in these patients.

Impotence
Although often not regarded as such, impotence may be an important problem in older hypertensive males. Various antihypertensive drugs are known for their effects on sexual function. Thiazide diuretics, α-adrenergic antagonists and β-adrenergic antagonists are best used with caution in patients with an active sexual life.

Benign prostatic hyperplasia
In recent years a new indication for α-adrenergic antagonists has emerged. In several studies α--adrenergic antagonists have slowed down the development of benign prostatic hyperplasia [91]. In a placebo-controlled study

obstructive complaints significantly decreased during doxazosin treatment [92].

Osteoporosis
Thiazide diuretics prescribed for the treatment of hypertension may have a preventive effect on osteoporosis and proximal femoral fractures [93]. Although it is too early to prescribe thiazide diuretics as a preventive measure for the development of osteoporosis, they may be preferred as antihypertensive drug in middle-aged and older women whenever they are judged to be equal to other antihypertensive drugs.

Final remarks

In the context of this chapter, the distinction between young and old hypertensives is an artificial one and therefore the approach of hypertensives with one concomitant illness is not really dependent of their age. The elderly, however, often have several diseases in one, making adequate treatment without causing side effects very difficult. In addition, available literature on hypertension and concomitant disease is relatively scant.

The problem of which antihypertensive drug to use, preferentially in the aged, remains unsolved. Because elderly people are less able to maintain homeostasis, they tend to be more prone to adverse effects, making close surveillance of any therapy mandatory. In any case, non-pharmacological treatment should be instituted first. Antihypertensive therapy can be individualized because of the wide array of available drugs. In this way it is possible to optimize the antihypertensive treatment without causing the incidence of side effects to increase.

Practical guidelines

Elderly patients need extra care with regard to explicitation, instruction and control. Only then, patient compliance can be optimal and antihypertensive treatment successful.

In general: Check whether the patient understands your information and instructions. Initiate antihypertensive treatment only when the diagnosis of hypertension is definite. Start antihypertensive treatment only after inventarisation of concomitant diseases and in the context of the cardiovascular risk profile. Start with non-pharmacological treatment; it is worthwhile trying. Wait sufficiently long enough to give non-pharmacological treatment a chance. When antihypertensive drugs are necessary, start at a lower dose than usual and increase the dose with smaller steps, under close surveillance of the patient. Try regimens with once-daily administration and avoid multi-

Table 5. Practical considerations

	diuretics	β-adrenergic antagonists	α-adrenergic antagonists	calcium-entry blockers	ACE-inhibitors
LVH	+	+	+	+	+
CHF	+ +	−	+	+‡	+ +
CAD	±	+ +	±	+	+
PVD	±	−†	±	+	+
OH	−	−	−	+	+
DM	−	−?	?	+	+ +
RF	+*	−?	±?	+	+**
COPD	±	−	+	+	±
MD	+	−?	−?	+	+
SD	−	−	−	+	+

LVH=	left ventricular hypertrophy	RF = renal failure
CHF=	congestive hear failure	COPD= chronic obstructive pulmonary disease
CAD=	coronary artery disease	
PVD=	peripheral vascular disease	MD = mental dysfunction
OH =	orthostatic hypotension	SD = sexual dysfunction
DM =	diabetes mellitus	PAA = partial agonistic activity

− = to avoid, ± = indifferent, + = allowed, + + = preferentially.
* loop diuretics.
† non-PAA.
‡ dihydriopyridines.
** low dose.

ple drug regimens. Always ask yourself what drug is contraindicated or less wanted and what drug may be of particular benefit.

Specific: Pharmacological antihypertensive treatment should be individualized. Titrate drugs on standing blood pressure to minimize orthostatic hypotension. Combine drugs with additive effects (different pharmacodynamic properties) or with counter-regulatory effects to minimize dose and side effects. In case of relevant concomitant diseases choose the antihypertensive drug according to present knowledge, as schematically depicted in Table 5.

References

1. The 1988 Joint National Committee. The 1988 report of the joint national committee on detection, evaluation and treatment of high blood pressure. Arch Intern Med 1988; **148**: 1023–38.
2. Kannel WB. Potency of vascular risk factors as the basis for antihypertensive therapy. Eur Heart J 1992; **13** (Suppl. G): 34–42.
3. Black HR. Nonpharmacological therapy for hypertension in the elderly. Geriatrics 1989; **44**: 20–9.

4. Applegate WB, Miller ST, Elam JT et al. Nonpharmacologic intervention to reduce blood pressure in older patients with mild hypertension. Arch Int Med 1992; **152**: 1162–6.
5. World Hypertension League. Physical exercise in the management of hypertension: A consensus statement by the World Hypertension League. J Hypertens 1991; **9**: 283–7.
6. Myers JB, Morgan TO. The effect of sodium intake on the blood pressure related to age and sex. Clin Exp Hypertens 1983; **5**: 99–118.
7. Klatsky AL, Friedman GD, Siegelaub AB, Gerard MJ. Alcohol consumption among white, black or oriental men and women. Kaiser–Permanente multiphasic health examination data. Am J Epidemiol 1977; **105**: 311–23.
8. Levy D. Left ventricular hypertrophy: Epidemiological insights from the Framingham study. Drugs 1988; **35** (Suppl. 35): 1–5.
9. Why HJF, Richardson PJ. Effect of carvedilol on left ventricular function and mass in hypertension. J Cardiovasc Pharmacol 1992; **19** (Suppl. 1): S50–S54.
10. Dahlöf B, Pennert K, Hansson L. Reversal of left ventricular hypertrophy in hypertensive patients: Meta-analysis of 109 treatment studies. Am J Hypertens 1992; **5**: 95–110.
11. Dahlöf B. Regression of cardiovascular structural changes: A preventive strategy. Clin Exp Hypertens A 1990; **12**: 877–96.
12. Nagano N, Iwatsubo H, Hata T, Mikami H, Ogihara T. Effects of antihypertensive treatment on cardiac hypertrophy and cardiac function in elderly hypertensive patients. J Cardiovasc Pharmacol 1991; **17** (Suppl. 2): S163–S165.
13. Van Hoof R, Staessen J, Fagard R, Thijs L, Amery A. The effect of antihypertensive treatment on electrocardiogram voltages in the EWPHE trial. J Cardiovasc Pharmacol 1991; **17** (Suppl. 2): S101–S104.
14. Schulman SP, Weiss JL, Becker LC et al. The effects of antihypertensive therapy on left ventricular mass in elderly patients. N Engl J Med 1990; **322**: 1350–6.
15. The SHEP Cooperative Research Group. Prevention of stroke by antihypertensive treatment in older persons with isolated systolic hypertension: Final results of the Systolic Hypertension in the Elderly Program (SHEP). JAMA 1991; **265**: 3255–64.
16. Cohn JN, Johnson G. Heart failure with normal ejection fraction: The V-HEFT Study. Circulation 1990; **81** (Suppl. 2): 48–53.
17. The SOLVD investigators. Effect of enalapril on survival in patients with reduced left ventricular ejection fraction and congestive heart failure. N Engl J Med 1991; **325**: 293–302.
18. Pfeffer MA, Braunwald E, Moye LA et al. Effect of captopril on mortality and morbidity in patients with left ventricular dysfunction after myocardial infarction. Results of the survival and ventricular enlargement trial. N Engl J Med 1992; **327**: 669–77.
19. The CONSENSUS Trial Study Group. Effects of enalapril on mortality in severe congestive heart failure: Results of the Cooperative North Scandinavian Enalapril Survival Study (CONSENSUS). N Engl J Med 1987; **316**: 1429–35.
20. Schwartz BM, Sackner-Bernstein J, Penn J et al. Which patients with congestive heart failure are most likely to show hemodynamic and functional improvement following long term beta blockade? J Am Coll Cardiol 1992; **19** (Suppl. A): 341.
21. Vanhoutte P, Amery A, Birkenhäger W et al. Serotonergic mechanisms in hypertension: Focus on the effect of ketanserin. Hypertension 1988; **11**: 111–33.
22. Jost S, Deckers JW, Nikutta P et al. Progression of coronary artery disease is dependent on anatomic location and diameter. J Am Coll Cardiol 1993; **21**: 1339–46.
23. Pfeffer MA, Lamas GA, Vaughan DE, Parisi AF, Braunwald E. Effect of captopril on progressive ventricular dilatation after anterior myocardial infarction. N Engl J Med 1988; **319**: 80–6.
24. Weber KT, Janicki JS. Angiotensin and the remodelling of the myocardium. Br J Clin Pharmacol 1989; **28** :141S–150S.
25. Cleland JG, Dargie HJ, Hodsman GP et al. Captopril in heart failure: A double blind controlled trial. Br Heart J 1984; **52**: 530–5.

26. Prevention of Atherosclerotic Complications with Ketanserin Trial Group. Prevention of atherosclerotic complications: Controlled trial of ketanserin. Br Med J 1989; **298**: 424–30.
27. Hachinsky V. Hypertension in acute ischemic strokes. Arch Neurol 1985; **42**: 1002.
28. Jansen PAF, Schulte BPM, Poels EFJ, Gribnau FWJ. Course of blood pressure after cerebral infarction and transient ischemic attack. Clin Neurol Neurosurg 1987; **89**: 243–6.
29. Gelmers HJ, Gorter K, De Weerdt CJ, Wiezer HJA. A controlled trial of nifedipine in acute ischemic stroke. N Engl J Med 1988; **318**: 203–7.
30. Burke V, Beilin H, German R et al. Postural fall in blood pressure in the elderly in relation to drug treatment and other lifestyle factors. Q J Med 1992; **304**: 583–91.
31. Clement DL, Duprez D. Effect of ketanserin in the treatment of patients with intermittent claudication: Results from 13 placebo-controlled parallel group studies. J Cardiovasc Pharmacol 1987; **10** (Suppl. 3): S89–S95.
32. Omoigui N, Dzau VJ. Differential effects of antihypertensive agents in experimental and human atherosclerosis. Am J Hypertens 1993; **6**: 30S–39S.
33. Henry PD. Calciumantagonists as anti-atherosclerotic agents. Arteriosclerosis 1990; **10**: 963–5.
34. Waters D, Lespérance J, Francetisch M et al. A controlled clinical trial to assess the effects of a calcium channel blocker on the progression of coronary atherosclerosis. Circulation 1990; **82**: 1940–53.
35. Lichtlén PR, Hugenholtz PG, Rafflenbeul W, Hecker H, Jost S, Deckers JW. Retardation of angiographic progression of coronary artery disease by nifedipine. Results of the International Nifedipine Trial on Anti-atherosclerotic Therapy (INTACT). Lancet 1990; **335**: 1109–13.
36. Kober G, Schneider W, Kaltenbach M. Can the progression of coronary sclerosis be influenced by calcium antagonists? J Cardiovasc Pharmacol 1989; **13** (Suppl. 4): S2–S6.
37. Furberg CD, Borhani NO, Byington RP, Gibbons ME, Sowers JR. Calcium antagonists and atherosclerosis: The Multicenter Isradipine/Diuretic Atherosclerosis Study. Am J Hypertens 1993; **6**: 24S–29S.
38. Thiery J, Stibbe W, Franz U, Müller B, Seidel D. Influence of ketanserin and flunarizin on the development of atherosclerosis in cholesterol-fed rabbits. 1986. (Abstract).
39. Williams RR, Hunt SC, Hopkins PN et al. Familial dyslipidemic hypertension: Evidence from 58 Utah families for a syndrome present in approximately 12% of patients with essential hypertension. JAMA 1988; **259**: 3579–86.
40. Papalia D, Casale P. Effect of nitrendipine in mild or moderate essential hypertensive subjects with type II diabetes. J Cardiovasc Pharmacol 1991; **18** (Suppl. 1): S98–S100.
41. Sheu WHH, Swislocki ALM, Hoffman B et al. Comparison of the effects of atenolol and nifedipine on glucose, insulin, and lipid metabolism in patients with hypertension. Am J Hypertens 1991; **4**: 199–205.
42. Schernthaner G, Sinzinger H, Siberbauer K, Freyter H, Mihlauser I, Kalman J. Vascular prostacyclin, platelet sensitivity to prostaglandines and platelet specific proteins in diabetes mellitus. Horm Metab Res 1981; Suppl. 11: 33–43.
43. Betz E, Kling D. The effect of calcium antagonists on intimal cell proliferation in atherogenesis. Ann NY Acad Sci 1988; **522**: 420.
44. Pollare T, Lithell H, Selinus I, Berne C. Sensitivity to insulin during treatment with atenolol and metoprolol: A randomized double-blind study of effects on carbohydrate and lipoprotein metabolism in hypertensive patients. Br Med J 1989; **298**: 1152–7.
45. Ferrari P, Rosman J, Weidmann P. Antihypertensive agents, serum lipoproteins and glucose metabolism. Am J Cardiol 1991; **67**: 26B–35B.
46. Nash DT, Schonfield G, Reeves RK, Black H, Weidler DJ. A double-blind trial to assess the efficacy of doxazosin, atenolol and placebo in patients with mild to moderate systemic hypertension. Am J Cardiol 1987; **59**: 88–90G.
47. Lithell HO, Pollare T, Berne C. Insulin sensitivity in newly detected hypertensive patients: Influence of captopril and other antihypertensive agents on insulin sensitivity and related biological parameters. J Cardiovasc Pharmacol 1990; **15** (Suppl. 5): S46–S52.

48. Anderson S, Rennke HG, Garcia DL, Brenner BM. Short and long term effect of antihypertensive treatment in the diabetic rat. Kidney Int 1989; **36**: 526–36.
49. Anderson S, Rennke HG, Brenner BM. Nifedipine versus fosinopril in uninephrectomized diabetic rats. Kidney Int 1992; **41**: 891–7.
50. Savage S, Miller LA, Schrier RW. The future of calcium channel blocker therapy in diabetes mellitus. J Cardiovasc Pharmacol 1991; **18** (Suppl. 1): S19–S24.
51. Mathiesen ER, Hommel E, Giese J, Parving HH. Efficacy of captopril in postponing nephropathy in normotensive insulin diabetic patients with microalbuminuria. Br Med J 1991; **303**: 81–7.
52. Brunner HR. ACE-inhibitors in renal disease. Kidney Int 1992; **42**: 463–79.
53. Parving HH, Smidt UM, Mathiesen ER, Hommel E. Ten years experience with antihypertensive treatment in diabetic nephropathy. Diabetologia 1991; **34** (Suppl. 2): A38.
54. Zucchelli P, Zuccala A, Borghi M et al. Long-term comparison between captopril and nifedipine in the progression of renal insufficiency. Kidney Int 1992; **42**: 452–8.
55. Weidmann P, Ferrier C, Saxenhofer H, Uehlinger DE, Trost BN. Serum lipoproteins during treatment with antihypertensive drugs. Drugs 1988; **35** (Suppl. 6): 118–34.
56. Staessen J, Amery A, Birkenhäger W et al. Is a high serum cholesterol level associated with larger survival in elderly hypertensives? J Hypertens 1990; **8**: 755–71.
57. Hunninghake DB. The effects of cardioselective vasodilating β-blockers on lipids. Am Heart J 1991; **121**: 1029–32.
58. Ruffolo RR, Boyle DA, Venuti RP, Lukas MA. Carvedilol (Kredex): A novel multiple action cardiovascular agent. Drugs Today 1991; **21**: 465–92.
59. Thaulow E, Nitter-Hauge S. Antihypertensive treament and blood lipids: Alpha-blockers. Scand J Clin Lab Invest 1990; **50** (Suppl. 199): 45–8.
60. Leren TP. Doxazosin increases low density cholesterol receptor activity. Acta Pharmacol Toxicol 1985; **56**: 269–72.
61. D'Eletto RD, Jawitt NB. Effect of doxazosin on cholesterol synthesis in cell culture. J Cardiovasc Pharmacol 1989; **13** (Suppl. 2): S1–S4.
62. Midtbo KA. Effects of long-term verapamil therapy on serum lipids and other metabolic parameters. Am J Cardiol 1990; **66** (Suppl. I): I13–I15.
63. Pool PE, Seagren SC, Salet AF, Skalland ML. Effects of diltiazem on serum lipids, exercise performance and blood pressure: Randomized, double-blind, placebo-controlled evaluation for systemic hypertension. Am J Cardiol 1985; **56** (Suppl. H): H86–H91.
64. Agner E. Antihypertensive therapy and blood lipids: ACE-inhibitors. Scand J Clin Lab Invest 1990; **50** (Suppl. 199): 55–9.
65. Shulman NB, Ford CE, Hall WD et al. Prognostic value of serum creatinine and effect of treament of hypertension on renal function: Results from the Hypertension Detection and Follow-up Program. Hypertension 1989; **13** (Suppl. I): 80–93.
66. Ruilope LM, Miranda B, Morales JM, Rodicio JL, Romero JC, Ray L. Converting enzyme inhibition in chronic renal failure. Am J Kidney Dis 1989; **13**: 120–6.
67. Kamper A-L, Strandgaard S, Leyssac PP. Effect of enalapril on the progression of chronic renal failure, A randomized controlled trial. Am J Hypertens 1992; **5**: 423–30.
68. Eliahou HE, Cohen D, Hellberg B et al. Effect of the calcium-channel blocker nisoldipine on the progression of chronic renal failure in man. Am J Nephrol 1988; **8**: 285–90.
69. Hall WD. Hemodynamic effects of antihypertensive agents in relation to kidney function. Choices Cardiol 1992; **6** (Suppl. 3): 10–1.
70. De Leeuw PW (EWPHE). Renal function in the elderly: Results from the European Working Party on High blood pressure in the Elderly trial. Am J Med 1991; **90** (Suppl. 3A): 45–9.
71. De Leeuw PW, Birkenhäger WH. Renal response to propanolol treatment in hypertensive humans. Hypertension 1982; **4**: 125–31.
72. Epstein M, Oster JR. Beta-blockers and renal function: A reappraisal. J Clin Hypertens 1985; **1**: 65–99.

73. Paillard F, Lantz B, Leviel F, Ardaillon R. Renal hemodynamic effects of tertalol in essential hypertension. Am J Nephrol 1986; **6** (Suppl. 2): 40–4.
74. Dupont AG, Van der Niepen P, Bossuyt AM, Jonckheer MH. Six RO. Nadolol in essential hypertension: Effect on ambulatory blood pressure, renal hemodynamics and cardiac function. Br J Clin Pharmacol 1985; **20**: 93–9.
75. Schmieder RE, Ruddell H, Schlebusch H et al. Impact of antihypertensive therapy with isradipine and metoprolol on early markers of hypertensive nephropathy. Am J Hypertens 1992; **5**: 318–21.
76. Apperloo AJ, De Zeeuw D, Sluiter HE et al. Differential effects of enalapril and atenolol on proteinuria and renal haemodynamics in non-diabetic renal disease. Br Med J 1991; **303**: 821–4.
77. Bauer JH. Adrenergic blocking agents and the kidney. J Clin Hypertens 1985; **3**: 199–208.
78. Rasmussen S, Nielsen PE. Blood pressure, body fluid volumes and glomerular filtration rate during treatment with labetolol in essential hypertension. Br J Clin Pharmacol 1981; **12**: 349–53.
79. Lin H, Young DB. The antihypertensive mechanism of verapamil: Alteration of GFR regulation. Hypertension 1988; **11**: 639–44.
80. Campbell DJ. Circulating and tissue angiotensin system. J Clin Invest 1987; **79**: 1–6.
81. Bianchi S, Bigazzi R, Baldari G et al. Microalbuminuria in patients with essential hypertension: Effects of an angiotensin converting enzyme inhibitor and of a calcium channel blocker. J Hypertens 1991; **4**: 291–6.
82. Rosenberg ME, Hostetter TH. Comparative effects of antihypertensives on proteinuria: Angiotensin-converting enzym inhibitor versus α-antagonist. Am J Kidney Dis 1991; **18**(4): 472–82.
83. Hannedouche T, Godin M, Fries D, Fillastre JP. Acute renal thrombosis induced by angiotensin-converting enzyme inhibitors in patients with renovascular hypertension. Nephron 1991; **57**: 231.
84. Starr JM, Whalley LJ, Inch S, Shering PA. Blood pressure and cognitive function in healthy old people. JAGS 1993; **41**: 753–6.
85. Cushman WC, Khatri I, Materson BJ et al. Treatment of hypertension in the elderly. Response of isolated systolic hypertension to various doses of hydrochlorothiazide: Results of a department of Veterans Affairs cooperative study. Arch Intern Med 1991; **151**: 1954–60.
86. Kalra L, Jackson SHD, Swift CG. Effect of antihypertensive treatment on psychomotor performance in the elderly. J Human Hypertens 1993; **7**: 285–90.
87. Dimsdale J, Newton R, Joist T. Neuropsychological side effects of beta blockers. Arch Intern Med 1989; **149**: 514–25.
88. Olajide S, Lader M. Psychotropic effects of enalapril maleate in normal volunteers. Psychopharmacology 1985; **86**: 374–6.
89. Currie D, Lewis RV, McDevitt DG et al. Central effects of the angiotensin-converting enzyme inhibitor captopril: I-Performance and subjective assessments of mood. Br J Clin Pharmacol 1990; **30**: 527–36.
90. McDevitt DG, Currie D, Nicholson AN et al. Central effects of the calcium antagonist nifedipine. Br J Clin Pharmacol 1991; **32**: 541–9.
91. Lepor H. Role of alpha-adrenergic blockers in the treatment of benign prostatic hyperplasia. Prostate 1990; **3** (Suppl.): 75–84.
92. Christensen MM, Bendix-Holme J, Rasmussen PC et al. Doxazosin treatment in patients with prostatic obstruction: A double-blind placebo-controlled study. Scand J Urol Nephrol 1993; **27**: 39–44.
93. Ray WA, Griffin MR, Downey W, Melton LJ. Long-term use of thiazide diuretics and risk of hip fractures. Lancet 1989; **i**: 687–90.

5. Therapeutic trials in elderly hypertensives: meta-analysis and implications for daily practice

R. VAN HOOF, L. THIJS, J. STAESSEN, R. FAGARD, H. CELIS, W. BIRKENHÄGER and A. AMERY

During the last years, several outcome trials in elderly hypertensive patients have been published.

The purpose of this paper is first to present a meta-analysis of these trials and second to try to answer a few questions related to our daily practice in elderly hypertensive patients based on the results of these trials.

A. META-ANALYSIS OF OUTCOME TRIALS IN ELDERLY HYPERTENSIVES

Introduction

From 1971 onwards, several prospective randomized outcome trials on anti-hypertensive drug treatment in elderly hypertensive patients have been published [1–11]. Four studies [1–3, 6] included younger as well as older patients, while seven studies [4, 5, 7–11] considered exclusively patients of 60 years and older. The sample sizes of the elderly patients in most of the individual studies may have been too small to detect a significant reduction in all-cause or cause-specific mortality! In addition, the generalizability of each of these studies is limited by the selection of the patients and by the specificity of the treatment protocol. Combining trials in a meta-analysis increases the power of the statistical analysis and allows us to examine the generalizability of the results to a more varied range of patients and treatment protocols. A more precise estimate of the magnitude of the true treatment effect may also be provided [12–17].

In a previous meta-analysis of five studies [3, 4, 6–8], Staessen et al. [18] have demonstrated a significant reduction in cardiovascular mortality (-28%, $p < 0.02$) and a similar tendency in all-cause mortality (-14%, $p = 0.07$). Since this meta-analysis, three more randomized therapeutic trials in elderly

Gastone Leonetti and Cesare Cuspidi (eds), Hypertension in the Elderly, 71–89
© 1994 *Kluwer Academic Publishers. Printed in the Netherlands*

hypertensive patients have been published. The Swedish Trial in Old Patients with Hypertension [10] (STOP-Hypertension) and the British Medical Research Council trial of hypertension in older adults [11] (MRC) included mainly patients with combined systolic and diastolic hypertension, whereas the Systolic Hypertension in the Elderly Program (SHEP) [9] recruited exclusively patients with isolated systolic hypertension (diastolic pressure <90 mmHg). The purpose of the present meta-analysis was to update the estimates of the magnitude of the treatment effect on all-cause and cause-specific mortality and on non-fatal cardiovascular events in elderly patients with systolic and diastolic hypertension. Because isolated systolic hypertension constitutes a separate pathophysiological entity, SHEP was not included in the meta-analysis, but will be discussed separately.

The methods used for the present meta-analysis have been described in detail by Thijs et al. [22].

Results of the meta-analysis

Selection of trials

A total of 11 published randomized studies, conducted between 1964 and 1992, were identified:

1. the trial by the US Veterans Administration Cooperative Study Group (VACS) [1],
2. the trial in stroke survivors by the Hypertension Stroke Cooperative Study Group (HSCS) [2],
3. the Hypertension Detection and Follow-up Program (HDFP) [3],
4. the Japanese study of mild hypertension in the aged by Kuramoto et al. (KURAMOTO) [4],
5. the study by Sprackling et al. [5],
6. the Australian Therapeutic Trial in Mild Hypertension (ATTMH) [6],
7. the European Working Party on High blood pressure in the Elderly trial (EWPHE) [7],
8. Coope and Warrender's trial on the treatment of hypertension in the elderly patients in primary care (COOPE) [8],
9. the Systolic Hypertension in the Elderly Program (SHEP) [9],
10. the Swedish Trial in Old Patients with Hypertension (STOP) [10],
11. the British Medical Research Council trial of treatment of hypertension in older adults (MRC) [11].

Three trials were not included in the meta-analysis. In one trial absolute figures of mortality and morbidity were not presented [5]. The SHEP trial, which included only patients with isolated systolic hypertension, was not considered in the combined analysis since isolated systolic hypertension is a different pathophysiological entity. The HDFP was excluded from the meta-analysis because this study did not compare active treatment with no or placebo treatment, but care in specialized centres with regular care.

Description of the trials included in the meta-analysis

The characteristics of the 8 trials considered in the meta-analysis concerning all-cause and cause-specific mortality are summarized in Table 1. The combined analysis included a total of 8701 elderly patients of whom 4395 belonged to the control groups and 4306 to the intervention groups. The number of patients randomized in each of the studies ranged from 81 in the trial by the US Veterans Administration Cooperative Study Group to 4396 in the MRC trial. Some trials included younger as well as older patients, but only the subgroup of patients above the age of 60 years was considered in the meta-analysis. One study had an open design, two a single-blind design and five a double-blind design.

The risk of experiencing a fatal event in the control group differed widely among trials and this may reflect the differences in selection and recruitment among the studies. Some studies recruited their patients via population screening, others via general practice, old people's homes, outpatient clinics or combinations of these. Also the entry criteria for the blood pressure, the goal of treatment and the antihypertensive drugs used to achieve the goal blood pressure varied from study to study (Table 1).

All-cause and cause-specific mortality

Absolute figures of mortality were available in 6 trials. Figure 1 illustrates that all-cause mortality tended to decrease in all these 6 trials except in the small Japanese trial by Kuramoto et al. The reduction in all-cause mortality reached statistical significance only in the STOP-Hypertension trial (-43%, 95% CI ranging from -61% to -15%). The overlap of the 95% confidence limits indicate that there was no significant difference between the results of the different trials. Why the reduction in all-cause mortality was significant in the STOP trial will be discussed later. Combining all 6 trials there was a tendency to a decrease in all-cause mortality by 9% ($-18\%-+1\%$), which was not statistically significant.

Active treatment did not significantly affect non-cardiovascular mortality in any of the studies. The Mantel–Haenszel estimate of the pooled treatment effect of $+11\%$ ($-6\%-+31\%$) was not statistically significant ($p = 0.24$; Figure 2). The STOP trial was the only trial which showed a tendency to a decrease in non-cardiovascular mortality and this explains in part the significant decrease in all-cause mortality in this trial.

In all studies, except the Japanese trial, cardiovascular mortality was lower in the intervention than in the control group. The difference between the 2 treatment groups was significant in the EWPHE study (-27%, $-45\%--2\%$) and in the STOP-Hypertension trial (-58%, $-76\%--27\%$). In the

Table 1. Characteristics of the studies or subgroups of patients considered in the meta-analysis

	VACSG [1]	HSCSG [2]	KURAMOTO [4]	ATTMH [6]
Sample size	81	200	91	582
Year of publication	1972	1974	1981	1981
Design	double-blind	double-blind	double-blind	single-blind
Age range (years)	60–75	60–75	60–90	60–69
Percentage women	0	NR	45	45
Follow-up (years)	NR	NR	4	4
Recruitment	out-patient clinics	out-patient clinics	old people's homes	population screening
First line treatment	– hydrochlorothiazide +reserpine – hydralozine hydrochloride	deserpine+ methylclotiazide	trichlormethiazide	chlorothiazide
Additional therapy	–	–	– reserpine – methyldopa – hydralazine	– or methyldopa or propranolol or pindolol – or hydralazine or clonidine
BP at entry (SBP/DBP)	free/90–114	140–220/90–115	160–200/90–110	<200/95–109
BP reduction (SBP/DBP)*	NR	NR	5/2	11/7
Lost to follow up (%)	NR	NR	6.6	2.1

	EWPHE [7]	COOPE [8]	STOP [10]	MRC [11]
Sample size	840	884	1627	4396
Year of publication	1985	1986	1991	1992
Design	double-blind	open	double-blind	single-blind
Age range (years)	60–96	60–79	70–84	65–74
Percentage women	70	70	63	58
Follow-up (years)	4.6	4.4	2	5.8

Recruitment	– out-patient clinics – population screening – sheltered housing or hospital wards	general practice	health centres	screening via registers of general practices
First line treatment	hydrochlorothiazide +triamterene	atenolol	– hydrochlorothiazide +amiloride – or atenolol or metoprolol or pindolol	– hydrochlorothiazide +amiloride – atenolol
Additional therapy	methyldopa	– bendrofluazide – methyldopa – any therapy	– or atenolol or metoprolol or pindolol – hydroclorothiazide +amiloride	– atenolol nifedipine – hydrochlorothiazide +amiloride nifedipine
BP at entry (SBP/DBP)	160–239/90–119	170–280/<120 or <280/105–120	180–230/90–120 or <180/105–120	160–209/<115
BP reduction (SBP/DBP)*	21/7	±16/±10†	22/9	±16/±7†
Lost to follow up (%)	15.2	NR	0	25‡

* Difference in BP reduction between the intervention and control group. In all studies, except the ATTMH, the blood pressure at 1 year is taken into account. In the ATTMH all blood pressure readings on the trial regimen are considered.

† Read from the figures.

‡ As defined in the paper. All-cause and cause-specific mortality is known in 97% of the patients in the EWPHE-trial and in all patients in the MRC-trial.

NR = not reported.

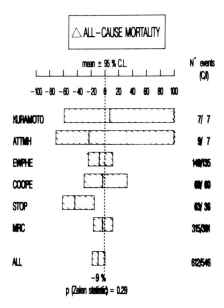

Figure 1. For each individual study, the percentage difference in all-cause mortality between the intervention and control group together with the 95% confidence interval (CI) of this difference. A negative sign indicates a decrease in mortality in the intervention group compared to the control group. The summary statistic calculated using the Mantel–Haenszel procedure is added at the bottom of the figures. A 95% CI that does not include zero corresponds to $p < 0.05$ for the comparison between the two treatment groups. For each study, the number of events (N° events) in the control and intervention group (C/I) are given. From Thijs et al. [22].

combined analysis, cardiovascular mortality decreased on average by 22% (−32%––10%) (Figure 3).

Treatment of hypertension tended to reduce coronary mortality in most trials, but this tendency was not significant in any of the individual studies. However, when all trial results were pooled, coronary mortality was reduced by 26% (−40%––9%), which was highly significant ($p = 0.004$; Figure 4).

In the 4 largest studies, cerebrovascular mortality was lower in the intervention group as compared with the control group. This decrease achieved statistical significance in the study by Coope and Warrender (−70%, −90%– −11%) and in the STOP-Hypertension trial (−73%, −91%––20%). Combining all trials, a significant decrease of 33% (−50%––9%) was observed (Figure 5).

Non-fatal events

Also non-fatal cardiovascular events were considered in the meta-analysis. However, the meta-analysis of the combined fatal and non-fatal cardiovascu-

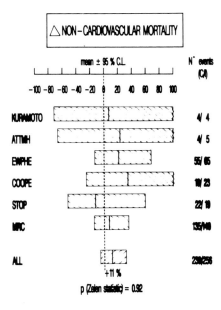

Figure 2. See legend to Figure 1 for non-cardiovascular mortality.

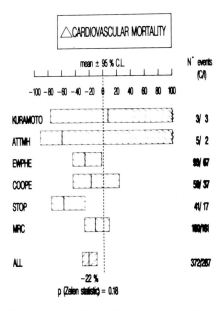

Figure 3. See legend to Figure 1 for cardiovascular mortality.

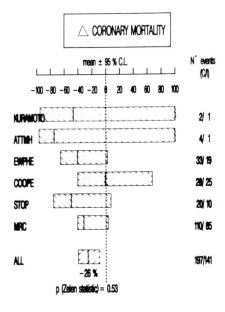

Figure 4. See legend to Figure 1 for coronary mortality.

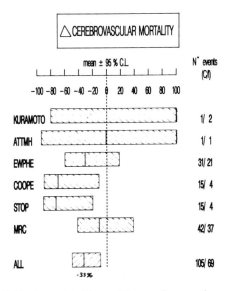

Figure 5. See legend to Figure 1 for cerebrovascular mortality.

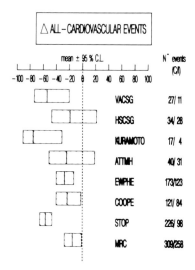

Figure 6. The percentage difference in all-cardiovascular events (fatal and non-fatal) between the intervention and control group together with the 95% confidence interval (CI) of this difference in 8 studies: 1. the trial by the US Veterans Administration Cooperative Study Group (VACSG); 2. the trial in stroke survivors by the Hypertension Stroke Cooperative Study Group (HSCSG); 3. the Japanese study of mild hypertension in the aged by Kuramoto et al. (KURAMOTO); 4. the Australian Therapeutic Trial in Mild Hypertension (ATTMH); 5. the European Working Party on High blood pressure in the Elderly trial (EWPHE); 6. Coope and Warrender's trial on the treatment of hypertension in the elderly patients in primary care (COOPE); 7. the Swedish Trial in Old Patients with hypertension (STOP); and 8. the British Medical Research Council trial of treatment of hypertension in older adults (MRC). A negative sign indicates a decrease in cardiovascular events in the intervention group. A 95% CI that does not include zero corresponds to $p < 0.05$ for the comparison between the two treatment groups. For each study, the number of events (N° events) in the control and intervention group (C/I) are given. The summary statistic is not presented because Zelen's test for homogeneity was highly significant ($p < 0.001$) indicating that there is no common underlying treatment effect.

lar events (Figure 6) showed a heterogenicity between the different trials. This suggests that the results of data pooled with the described method, must be interpreted with caution. The heterogeneity of the results between the different trials can be explained on the basis of differences in:

– recruitment of patients,
– treatment modalities such as differences in drugs, treatment regimen, etc.,
– treatment goals,
– statistical analyses of the results,
– endpoint criteria.

Especially the latter may differ largely from one trial to another when non-fatal events are considered. Coronary events may include myocardial infarction but also angina pectoris. Heart failure may include different stages of the disease. Cerebrovascular events may include completed stroke, but also transient ischaemic attacks and RINDs (reversible ischaemic neurological deficits). Also increase in blood pressure is considered as a non-fatal cardio-vascular event in some trials. Therefore we decided not to present pooled results of non-fatal cardiovascular events in this meta-analysis.

B. IMPLICATIONS FOR DAILY PRACTICE IN ELDERLY PATIENTS WITH SYSTOLO-DIASTOLIC HYPERTENSION

In the second part of this paper an attempt will be made to answer on the basis of the results of these outcome trials a few questions which are often raised in the daily practice of elderly hypertensive patients.

Why should we treat elderly hypertensive patients?

In a particular patient, treatment may be indicated because of the presence of signs of hypertension which are likely to be relieved by drug therapy. They include signs or symptoms of congestive heart failure, angina pectoris, hypertensive headache, etc. Treatment of these patients may improve their quality of life, which by itself may constitute an indication for drug therapy.

How should we approach the symptomless elderly ? What can we expect from drug therapy?

Except for one trial, all-cause mortality was not significantly reduced in the separate trials. Pooling the data suggests a 9% decrease but this difference was just short of statistical significance. So we cannot guarantee that drug treatment will prolong life of the patients.

On the other hand, fatal cardiovascular complications were significantly reduced and this seems a solid basis for the indication of drug therapy.

However, we should be aware that therapy will induce side-effects.

In the MRC trial [23] the diuretic treatment group showed an increased withdrawal rate for gout, skin disorders, muscle cramps, nausea and dizziness. In the beta-blocker group an increased withdrawal rate was observed, because of Raynaud's phenomenon, dyspnoe, lethargy and headache. Although the MRC trial was not a double-blind trial, the data strongly suggest that the quality of life was decreased in some patients.

Based on the EWPHE data, Fletcher et al. [24] considered the benefit and risk of therapy, by calculating the difference between the placebo and actively treated group; the data were expressed per 1000 patient-years. On the benefit side there was a significant decrease in fatal cardiac events (−11%), non-fatal stroke (−11%) and severe congestive heart failure (−8%). On the other hand there was an increase in gout (+4%), probably caused by the diuretics, and also an increase in dry mouth (+124%) and

CARDIOVASCULAR STUDY TERMINATING
EVENTS - R

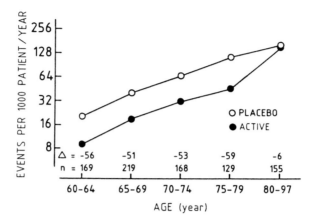

Figure 7. The number of cardiovascular study terminating events per 1000 patient years is shown for the 5 age subgroups on randomized treatment (R). Delta is the event reduction between the active and placebo treated subgroup. Event rates are represented on a logarithmic scale. (From Amery et al. [25].)

diarrhoea (+71%), probably caused by methyldopa. Although treatment can cause side-effects, on average the advantages of treatment seem to exceed the disadvantages in this EWPHE trial. Thus, drug treatment seems indicated in elderly patients with combined systolic and diastolic hypertension.

Upto which age should we treat our patients with systolo-diastolic hypertension?

We would like to consider not only the chronological age but also the biological age. However, the latter is more difficult to quantify and was not considered in any of these trials. Therefore we have to stick to the chronological age.

As can be seen from Table 1, the large MRC trial admitted patients in the age range from 65 to 75 years and only 3 trials admitted patients above age 80. The relationship between treatment effect and age will therefore be considered in more detail, in an attempt to answer this question.

In a subgroup analysing the EWPHE trial, using a Cox regression model, Amery et al. [25] confirmed that cardiovascular mortality was decreased by therapy and that there was a significant interaction between the treatment effect and age. This is illustrated in Figure 7: in the age group upto 79 there

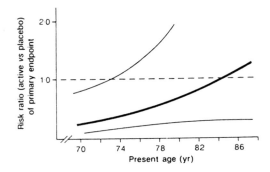

Figure 8. Relationship between age and the odds of experiencing a primary endpoint in the STOP-trial. Point estimates and 95% confidence limits are presented. (From Dahlöf et al. [10].)

is a tendency to less cardiovascular complications in the actively treated group, but this advantage is lost above age 80.

In the STOP-Hypertension trial [10] this relationship was also considered, as illustrated in Figure 8. This shows that the upper 95% confidence limits crosses the zero line around age 73, suggesting that above this age the advantage of therapy cannot be certified with confidence, the latter may be due to the lower number of patients admitted in the high age groups.

Summarizing the available data it seems advisable to start treatment in the hypertensive patients up to age 75. Whether therapy is also indicated at higher age in symptom-free patients without cardiovascular complications is less certain and a trial in this age group is now under consideration [26].

A problem which often emerges during the care of elderly hypertensives is whether we should stop antihypertensive drug therapy when the patients reach the age of 75 years. This was not specifically addressed in any of the trials and therefore no scientifically based answer can be provided. The following attitude may seem logical. We may first try to remember why antihypertensive drug therapy was started in this patient. If this reason is still present, continuation of therapy seems logical. If the patient has a symptomless uncomplicated hypertension some physicians will just continue therapy, while other physicians will try to decrease the dose of the drugs and follow the patient. If no symptoms appear one may continue the treatment at lower doses or even stop antihypertensive drug therapy.

From which diastolic blood pressure on is treatment indicated?

Blood pressure is more unstable in elderly than in younger patients and therefore repeated measurements at several occasions are necessary before deciding to treat a particular patient. This was also done in the trials.

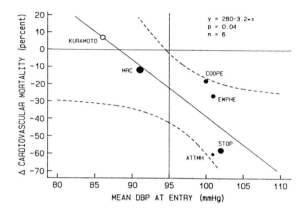

Figure 9. For each individual study, the percentage difference in cardiovascular mortality between the intervention and control group versus the mean diastolic blood pressure at randomisation. The size of each dot is proportional to the number of patients included in the study. The full line indicates the regression line and the dotted lines the 95% confidence limits of the mean. The regression line was weighted for the number of patients in each study (From Thijs et al. [22].]

The range of diastolic entry criteria varied widely between the several trials and this is reflected by the difference in the average diastolic pressure in each trial. Figure 9 shows for each of the trials the average diastolic blood pressure at entry in the trial and the decrease in cardiovascular mortality during the trial, comparing the placebo and active treatment group. The regression was weighted according to the number of patients admitted in each trial: the MRC trial which was by far the largest trial had the biggest weight, while the weight was smaller for the Kuramoto trial and the elderly section of the Australian trial (ATTMH). The regression line shows a negative correlation between the change in cardiovascular mortality and the entry diastolic pressure. In the STOP-trial with the highest average entry diastolic pressure, the decrease in cardiovascular mortality was most pronounced; the reduction was less profound in those trials where the entry diastolic blood pressure was lower.

Such a correlation does not proof per se a causal relationship; indeed several confounding factors could influence this relationship such as age, systolic blood pressure, differences in recruitment and treatment strategies in the different trials, and possibly others. It is also not definitely established whether the same relationship holds when individual patients are considered. A pooled analysis on the individual patients of all trials is indicated since analysis within each trial separately may lack the power to explore the possible influence of the entry blood pressure on the effect of treatment.

For the time being, the data show that the benefit of treatment in terms

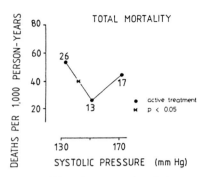

Figure 10. All-cause mortality, per 1000 patient years, in relation to systolic blood pressure on treatment in the actively treated patients of the EWPHE trial. The numbers indicate the number of deaths per 1000 patient years in each of the three thirds. (From Staessen et al. [27].)

of reduction in cardiovascular mortality, is not established in the studies when the entry diastolic pressure is below 95 mmHg.

What should be the goal blood pressure?

The overall goal of antihypertensive therapy should of course be to reduce morbidity and mortality and improve the quality of life.

One may however try to establish an intermediate goal based on the blood pressure. In the several trials the goal diastolic blood pressure varied widely: reduction of blood pressure below 105, 95, 90 and even below 80 mmHg. The goal systolic pressure was below 170, 160 and below 150 mmHg in some trials. The trial results have shown that the goal pressures were achieved in a large number of the patients and that this was accompanied by a reduction in cardiovascular morbidity. The question is, however, which is the optimal pressure to be achieved?

Not one trial looked specifically at this question. The HDFP [3] showed that stepped care (with more pressure reduction) was more efficient than regular care (with less pressure reduction) in preventing cardiovascular and all-cause mortality. However, the stepped-care group was different from the regular-care not only in the level of blood pressure reduction but also other measures of care were better administered in the former group. So we cannot conclude that the better prognosis in the stepped-care group was only due to the lower pressure. We therefore have to rely for the moment on post hoc analyses.

In an attempt to reach a better definition of the goal pressure we [27] analysed in the EWPHE data the relationship between the mortality and the systolic blood pressure during therapy (see Figure 10). The data show a U-shaped curve with the lowest mortality in the tertile with a systolic pressure around 150 mmHg and higher mortality (for all-cause, cardiovascular as well as non-cardiovascular) at a higher and lower systolic blood pressure level. This retrospective analysis suggests that a goal systolic blood pressure of 150 mmHg may be optimal. One should realise, however, that the increased mortality at lower systolic pressure (around 130) is not necessarily caused by an excessive blood pressure reduction. A U-shaped curve could also be observed in the placebo treated group [27], which strongly suggests that it was not drug induced; the patients with higher pressures (170 mmHg or more) may have been at higher risk because of the higher pressures and the patients with the lowest pressures may have been at higher risk because of other disease. Indeed, the most pronounced decreases in body weight and haemoglobin concentration tended to occur in the patients in the lowest thirds of systolic and diastolic blood pressure during treatment [27].

To define a goal pressure one should plan a trial specifically aimed at this and try to reduce the pressure to different levels in various groups and then consider the outcome in these groups. Results of such trials are not yet available.

Can we extrapolate from the patients studied in these trials to the elderly hypertensive population at large?

Except for the small Kuramoto trial [4], none of the trials were performed in Asia or Africa.

From a theoretical point of view, it may therefore be premature to extrapolate from the published trials to the African and Asian elderly hypertensive population. In addition, both in Japan, China and Africa, the nature of hypertensive cardiovascular complications is different from the complications in most Western countries: stroke being a relative more frequent complication than coronary events in the African and Asian populations. Thus extrapolation from these data to the latter populations may be premature.

Can we extrapolate the results of the intervention trials to the elderly hypertensive population at large in the Western countries? From a theoretical point of view, the results can only be extrapolated to a given defined population, if the trial was performed on a representative sample of this population. In none of the trials this was done. This was not the case, even the trials in which some screening of the population was performed.

However, although recruitment was different in the several trials (see Table 1) there is no indication that the outcome was different when the patients were recruited from different sources, other factors such as age and pressure being equal. It seems therefore acceptable to extrapolate the results of the trials to the elderly population at large in western countries at least within the age and pressure limits described above.

Which is the first drug of choice in elderly hypertensive patients?

In some hypertensive patients, there may be a specific indication for therapy which will also justify a specific drug therapy. For instance, in hypertensive patients with angina pectoris, beta-blockers and also calcium entry blockers will often be considered as the first drug of choice if there are no contra-indications. If the patients present signs or symptoms of congestive heart failure, diuretics and converting enzyme inhibitors may be the first drugs of choice.

Many elderly hypertensive patients do not present a specific indication for therapy, except for their high pressure: they have symptomless, uncomplicated hypertension. What are the first drugs of choice for these patients? In the latter patients the goal of therapy is not to relieve certain signs or symptoms, because, by definition, these patients are symptom-free. The goal of treatment is also not to reduce blood pressure, but the ultimate goal should be to reduce morbidity and mortality while improving the quality of life.

Most newer antihypertensive drugs have not been tested as first line drugs in these trials; thus we do not know whether calcium entry blockers, converting enzyme inhibitors, alpha-blockers or potassium channel openers are effective, as first line drugs, in reducing cardiovascular morbidity and mortality. Calcium entry blockers are being used in the Syst-Eur trial [20], as first line drugs. As long as the results of this and similar trials are not available, it seems wise to use mainly diuretics or beta-blockers as first line drugs, if there are no specific contra-indications. Indeed diuretics were shown to be effective in the Australian [6] and the EWPHE [7] trial and beta-blockers in Coope's trial [8].

In the STOP-trial [10] beta-blockers or diuretics were used as first line drugs and the therapy was overall effective in reducing all-cause mortality. Unfortunately, there was no stratification for diuretics and beta-blockers in this trial, so we do not know the relative effectiveness of the two classes of drugs.

In the MRC trial in elderly [11] diuretics and beta-blockers were also used as first line drugs and there was a stratification for diuretic or beta-blocker therapy. The results indicate that the favourable effects of drug therapy were seen in the diuretic and not in the beta-blocker treated group. It seems premature, however, to conclude from this single trial that only diuretics should be used as first line drugs in the treatment of elderly hypertensive patients. Indeed it is still possible that this was a chance finding. In addition the trial was single-blind and it is likely that quite some patients on beta-blockers were withdrawn because of slight bradycardia; these patients may have benefited most from the antihypertensive effect of the beta-blocker.

Furthermore one should not forget that in Coope's trial [8], where beta-blockers were used as first line drugs, there was a significant reduction in cerebrovascular mortality.

Thus, for the time being, diuretics and beta-blockers are the recommended first line drugs in the treatment of these patients.

Treatment of patients with isolated systolic hypertension (ISH)

Systolic hypertension is a major risk factor in elderly hypertensives and in some studies even more than diastolic hypertension [21]. Can we expect reduction of cardiovascular morbidity and mortality by drug treatment of these patients with ISH?

Three trials have been initiated limited to patients with ISH and a post hoc analysis of subgroups of two other trials is available.

In the post hoc analysis of the ISH patients of the Coope trial [8] and the EWPHE trial [7] there was no significant difference in cardiovascular mortality. These subgroups were however small: there were only 12 deaths in the intervention arms of the ISH subgroup of both trials.

The SHEP trial [9] was a major, randomized, double-blind, placebo-controlled trial, where 4736 patients with ISH were randomized. In the active treatment group chlorthalidone (12.5–25 mg) was the first step in therapy, followed by atenolol or reserpine. There was no significant decrease in all-cause mortality, non-cardiovascular mortality, cardiovascular mortality, stroke or coronary mortality.

There was, however, a significant decrease in the active treatment group in non-fatal stroke (96 versus 149 cases), non-fatal myocardial infarction (50 versus 74 cases), and left-ventricular failure (48 versus 108 cases).

In interpreting the results of this trial one should keep in mind that the patients were highly selected: only 1% of the screened patients was randomized while the prevalence of the ISH in these populations must be around 10%. All patients with major disease were excluded leading to a rather low mortality, even in the placebo treated group [19]. The outcome of the stroke patients is unclear: there were 149 non-fatal strokes, but only 14 fatal strokes; the outcome of the non-fatal strokes after a few weeks or months is not reported.

Because of these and other comments [19] and since the results of only one major trial on ISH is known, it may be premature to recommend drug therapy for the patients with ISH at large. We would prefer to wait for the results of two other major trials in patients with ISH, which are in progress, namely the Syst-Eur trial [20] in Europe and a similar trial in China: the Syst-Chin [28].

Conclusion

A meta-analysis is presented of 8 therapeutic trials in elderly hypertensive patients. In an intention-to-treat analysis, cardiovascular mortality was decreased on average by 22% (95% confidence interval ranging from −32% to −10%). This decrease was explained by both a reduction in coronary mortality by 26% (−40%−−9%) and in cerebrovascular mortality by 33% (−50%−−9%).

The effectiveness of therapy in terms of reducing cardiovascular mortality is not established with confidence in the trials where the diastolic blood pressure at randomization is below 95 mmHg or in the patients above 75 years of age.

A goal blood pressure is not definitively established but a reduction of the systolic blood pressure to about 150 mmHg may be optimal.

Extrapolation of the trial results to the elderly population with systolo-diastolic hypertension at large seems acceptable for the western population, but may be premature for the Asian and African elderly.

Beta-blockers and especially diuretics are recommended as the first line drugs in the elderly patients with symptomless, uncomplicated hypertension, since the effectiveness of other drugs in reducing morbidity and mortality is not yet established.

Recommendation for treatment of symptomless patients with isolated systolic hypertension may be premature. The ongoing Syst-Eur and Syst-Chin trials may provide further information.

References

1. Veterans Administration Cooperative Study Group on Anti-hypertensive Agents. Effects of treatment on morbidity in hypertension. Circulation 1972; **45**: 991–1004.
2. Hypertension–Stroke Cooperative Study Group. Effect of antihypertensive treatment on stroke recurrence. JAMA 1974; **229**: 409–418.
3. Hypertension Detection and Follow-up Program Cooperative Group. Five-year findings of the Hypertension Detection and Follow-up Program: II Mortality by race-sex and age. JAMA 1979; **242**: 2572–7.
4. Kuramoto K, Matsushita S, Kuwajima I, Murakawi M. Prospective study on the treatment of mild hypertension in the aged. Jpn Heart J 1981; **22**: 75–85.
5. Sprackling ME, Mitchell JRA, Short AH, Watt G. Blood pressure reduction in the elderly: A randomized controlled trial of methyldopa. Br Med J 1981; **283**: 1151–3.
6. Management Committee. Treatment of mild hypertension in the elderly: A study initiated and administered by the National Heart Foundation of Australia. Med J Aust 1981; **2**: 398–402.
7. Amery A, Birkenhäger W, Brixko R et al. Mortality and morbidity results from the European Working Party on high blood pressure in the elderly trial. Lancet 1985; **i**: 1349–54.
8. Coope J, Warrender TS. Randomised trial of treatment of hypertension in elderly patients in primary care. Br Med J 1986; **293**: 1145–51.
9. SHEP Cooperative Research Group. Prevention of stroke by antihypertensive drug treatment in older persons with isolated systolic hypertension: Final results of the Systolic Hypertension in the Elderly Program (SHEP). JAMA 1991; **265**: 3255–64.
10. Dahlöf B, Lindholm LH, Hansson L, Schersten B, Ekbom T, Wester PO. Morbidity and mortality in the Swedish Trial in Old Patients with Hypertension (STOP-Hypertension). Lancet 1991; **338**: 1281–5.

11. MRC Working Party. Medical Research Council trial of treatment of hypertension in older adults: Principal results. Br Med J 1992; **304**: 405–12.
12. Light RJ, Pillemer DB. Summing up: The science of reviewing research. Cambridge: Harvard University Press 1984.
13. Hedges LV, Olkin I. Statistical methods for meta-analysis. San Diego: Academic Press Inc 1985.
14. Thompson SG, Pocock SJ. Can meta-analysis be trusted? Lancet 1991; **338**: 1127–30.
15. Sacks HS, Berrier J, Reitman D, Ancona-Berk VA, Chalmers TC. Meta-analyses of randomized controlled trials. N Engl J Med 1987; **316**: 450–5.
16. L'Abbe KA, Detsky AS, O'Rourke K. Meta-analysis in clinical research. Ann Intern Med 1987; **107**: 224–33.
17. Bulpitt CJ. Meta-analysis. Lancet 1988; **i**: 93–4.
18. Staessen J, Fagard R, Van Hoof R, Amery A. Mortality in various intervention trials in elderly hypertensive patients: A review. Eur Heart J 1988; **9**: 215–22.
19. Staessen J, Fagard R, Amery A. Isolated systolic hypertension in the elderly: Implications of SHEP for clinical practice and for ongoing trials. J Hum Hypertens 1991; **5**: 469–74.
20. Amery A, Birkenhäger W, Bulpitt CJ et al. Syst-Eur: A multicentre trial on the treatment of isolated systolic hypertension in the elderly: Objectives, protocol, and organization. Aging 1991; **3**: 287–302.
21. Staessen J, Dekempeneer L, Fagard R et al. Treatment of isolated systolic hypertension in the elderly. J Cardiovasc Pharmacol 1991; **18** (Suppl. 1): S34–S40.
22. Thijs L, Fagard R, Lijnen P, Staessen J, Van Hoof R, Amery A. A meta-analysis of outcome trials in elderly hypertensives. J Hypertens 1992; **10**: 1103–9.
23. Medical Research Council Working Party on Mild to Moderate Hypertension: Adverse reactions to bendrofluazide and propranol for the treatment of mild hypertension. Lancet 1981; **ii**: 539–43.
24. Fletcher A, Amery A, Birkenhäger W et al. Risks and benefits in the trial of the European Working Party on High Blood Pressure in the Elderly. J Hypertens 1991; **9**: 225–30.
25. Amery A, Birkenhäger W, Brixko R et al. Efficacy of antihypertensive drug treatment according to age, sex, blood pressure, and previous cardiovascular disease in patients over the age of 60. Lancet 1986; **ii**: 589–92.
26. Bulpitt C. Personal communication.
27. Staessen J, Bulpitt C, Clement D et al. Relationship between mortality and treated blood pressure in elderly patients with hypertension: Report of the European Working Party on High Blood Pressure in the Elderly. Br Med J 1989; **298**: 1552–6.
28. Liu L. Personal communication.

6. Lessons from STOP-Hypertension

TORD EKBOM, LARS H. LINDHOLM, LENNART HANSSON,
BJÖRN DAHLÖF, ERLAND LINJER, BENGT SCHERSTÉN and
PER-OLOV WESTER

Introduction

The original ideas and plans for a major Swedish study on antihypertensive treatment in elderly patients were conceived in the early 1980s. At that time, it was well established that high blood pressure was closely correlated with increased morbidity and mortality from cardiovascular diseases in middle-aged people [1, 2]. For "younger elderly", up to the age of 70–75, some studies have demonstrated the value of antihypertensive treatment in reducing cardiovascular events [3, 4]. However, these results were mainly based on subgroup analyses and there have been no studies especially designed to evaluate the effects of pharmacological treatment of hypertension in patients aged 70 and above. For these reasons, the Swedish Trial in Old Patients with Hypertension (STOP-Hypertension) was set up and conducted under the supervision of the Swedish Hypertension Society in order to investigate the value of antihypertensive treatment in "old elderly" hypertensives.

Aim

The primary aim of STOP-Hypertension was to investigate whether elderly hypertensive men and women, aged 70–84 years, would benefit from antihypertensive therapy, compared to placebo in terms of reduced cardiovascular morbidity and mortality [5–8]. Secondary aims were to assess the effects of antihypertensive treatment on congestive heart failure, transient ischaemic attacks, angina pectoris, total mortality, and metabolic and subjective side-effects.

Gastone Leonetti and Cesare Cuspidi (eds), Hypertension in the Elderly, 91–101
© 1994 *Kluwer Academic Publishers. Printed in the Netherlands*

Study design

STOP-Hypertension was a multicentre study carried out at 116 health centres (out of 846) throughout Sweden, where hypertensive men and women aged 70–84 years were randomly allocated double-blind administration of active hypertensive therapy or placebo. The entry criteria were that on three separate occasions the systolic blood pressure was 180 mmHg, or above, with a diastolic blood pressure of at least 90 mmHg, or that the diastolic pressure was above 105 mmHg irrespective of the systolic blood pressure during a 1-month placebo run-in phase in previously untreated patients. The run-in phase was preceded by a 1–6-month washout period in previously treated patients.

Reasons for exclusion were a supine blood pressure above 230 mmHg systolic and/or 120 mmHg diastolic; isolated systolic hypertension (180 mmHg or higher with a diastolic blood pressure below 90 mmHg); orthostatic hypotension (more than 30 mmHg fall in systolic blood pressure on standing); contraindications to any of the drugs; a myocardial infarction or a stroke during the previous 12 months; angina pectoris requiring treatment with drugs other than nitrate preparations; other severe or incapacitating illnesses; or unwillingness to take part.

Blood pressure was measured by the same observer (nurse or doctor) for each patient throughout the study, after 5 min of recumbent rest and after 1 min of standing, by means of a mercury sphygmomanometer. The standard cuff bladder dimensions were 12×35 cm, but larger (15×43 cm) or smaller (9×25 cm) cuffs were used in patients with arm circumferences above 32 cm or below 22 cm, respectively. Disappearance of the Korotkoff sounds was recorded as the diastolic blood pressure. The average value of two recordings in the supine position, measured to the nearest 2 mmHg, was the main blood pressure variable upon which inclusion, changes in dosage, and so on, were determined.

Treatment consisted of Tenormin® 50 mg (atenolol), Moduretic® mite (hydrochlorothiazide 25 mg plus amiloride 2.5 mg, HCTZ + Am), Seloken® ZOC 100 mg (metoprolol CR), or Viskén® 5 mg (pindolol). All drugs were given once daily. If the supine blood pressure was 160 mmHg systolic and/or 95 mmHg diastolic, or above, after at least 2 months of treatment or at any later point during the study, the diuretic was added to the beta-blockers or vice versa. Each centre was free to choose any of the four basic regimens, which then had to be maintained throughout the study. Placebo tablets were identical in shape, taste, and colour to the active medication. If supine blood pressure exceeded 230/120 mmHg (and/or) on two subsequent visits the patient was changed to open antihypertensive treatment. After a non-fatal end-point, a patient could continue on double-blind treatment.

Recruitment took place between 14 November 1985 and 31 October 1990. The number of patients recruited was 1627, of whom 812 (mean age 75.7, SD 3.7) were randomly allocated to active treatment and 815 (mean age

75.6, SD 3.7) to placebo. When the trial was prematurely terminated it comprised 3390 patient-years of observation, with an average follow-up of 25 months regarding primary end-points.

The study had been approved by all ethical committees in Sweden and the National Board of Health and Welfare. It was carried out in accordance with the Declaration of Helsinki. Data auditing was performed in accordance with the recommendations of the US Food and Drug Administration on 10 randomly selected centres by an independent reviewer. That survey found no deviation from the study protocol of any kind that could affect the main purpose of the trial and that the study had been carried out in a scientifically correct manner. Accordingly its final results should be reliable.

The study was terminated on 8 April 1991 on the advice of the Safety Committee due to the increasing difference in endpoints between patients on treatment and placebo. Subsequently the investigators were advised that all blinded medication should be discontinued. All surviving patients were recalled and examined at the end of the study. No patient was lost to follow-up.

End-points were evaluated by an independent end-point committee, unaware of the patients' treatment or blood pressure. Their evaluation was based on medical records, death certificates, and necropsy reports, as appropriate. Primary end-points were stroke, myocardial infarction, and other cardiovascular death.

The pilot study

The main study was preceded by a 1-year pilot study in 31 centres, with the purpose of evaluating the logistic aspects, including the feasability of the study protocol, the possibilities of recruiting patients, and the percentage of screened patients that could be randomized [6]. During this period the centres consecutively registered all patients aged 70–84 years and in total 4668 patients were screened; 45% were found not to be hypertensive; 13.5% had an untreated supine blood pressure equal to or above 180/105 mmHg, and 41.5% were treated for hypertension, i.e. 55% were 'hypertensive'. Of the screened population 10% started a run-in/washout period. The reasons for not starting a run-in/washout period are given in Table 1. When the pilot study was concluded, 89 patients (1.9% of the screened population) had been randomized and 66 patients (1.4%) were still in the pipe-line of run-in/washout phase. After the pilot study the time-consuming consecutive screening procedures were not obligatory. For this reason there are no exact figures for the total 'screened' population that yielded the final cohort of 1627 patients.

Table 1. Reasons why 90% of the screened patients in the pilot study (*n* = 4,668) did not start the run-in/washout period

Reason	%
Orthostatic blood pressure fall (>30 mmHg systolic)	0.4
Blood pressure >230/120 mmHg (and/or)	0.9
Stroke within 12 months	1.0
Myocardial infarction within 12 months	1.4
Severe mental disability	1.8
Serum creatinine >200 mmol/L	2.7
Contra-indications for treatment with beta-blockers and diuretics	3.3
Angina pectoris needing treatment beyond nitrates	3.3
Isolated systolic hypertension (>180/<90 mmHg)	3.7
Severe physical disability	3.7
Unwillingness to participate	7.8
Treatment with beta-blockers or diuretics for reasons other than hypertension	12.8
Other reasons (including missing data)	2.1
Not hypertensive	45.0

Statistics

All analyses were based on the intention-to-treat principle. For continuous variables 95% confidence intervals (95% CI) were determined by use of the *t*-distribution, i.e. the variables were assumed to be normally distributed. Confidence intervals for proportions are calculated by usual normal distribution approximations. All tests are two-sided.

The study size of STOP-Hypertension was based on the assumption that 30% of strokes and myocardial infarctions would be fatal, that the risk reduction would be 1.75 % per mmHg reduction in systolic blood pressure, and that active treatment would lower systolic blood pressure by 20 mmHg more than would placebo. Based on Swedish mortality statistics it was calculated that 6000 patient-years would be needed to show a significant reduction in primary end-points with a statistical power of 90% at the significance level of 0.05 (by a two-tailed test). The analysis of total primary end-points was made on the first end-point that happened to an individual patient.

Patients

The major baseline characteristics of the 1627 patients in the trial are given in Table 2 [8]. Due to the exclusion criteria applied to the potential study patients, those randomized were in relatively good health. This was reflected by the fact that the study population compared to the Swedish normal population, taking sex, current age and calendar year into consideration, had a lower mortality. In the placebo group 63 deaths occurred while 90.4 deaths had been expected ($p < 0.01$) and in the actively treated patients 36 deaths

Table 2. Baseline characteristics of patients in STOP-Hypertension by treatment group

	Placebo ($n = 815$)	Active ($n = 812$)
Mean (SD) age in years	75.7 (3.7)	75.6 (3.7)
No (%) aged		
70–74 year	351 (43%)	363 (45%)
75–79 year	331 (41%)	313 (39%)
≥80 year	133 (16%)	136 (17%)
No (%) female	509 (63%)	510 (63%)
Mean (SD) body mass index (kg/m²)	26.5 (3.8)	26.7 (3.9)
Mean (SD) blood pressure (mmHg)		
Supine systolic	195 (14)	195 (14)
Supine diastolic	102 (7)	102 (7)
Standing systolic	188 (17)	187 (17)
Standing diastolic	104 (9)	104 (9)
Patients (%) included by type		
of hypertension		
<180/105 mmHg	7%	8%
≥180/90–104 mmHg	60%	62%
≥180/105 mmHg	33%	30%
Mean (SD) heart rate (bpm)		
Supine	76 (11)	77 (11)
Standing	82 (11)	82 (11)
No (%) previously treated*	416 (51%)	438 (54%)
No (%) smokers*	58 (7%)	69 (9%)
Previous stroke[†‡]	36 (4.5%)	32 (4%)
Previous myocardial infarction[†‡]	16 (2%)	17 (2.1%)
Diabetes mellitus[‡]	58 (7.2%)	69 (8.6%)

* Less than 6 months before run-in period.
[†] More than twelve months before randomization.
[‡] Based on placebo $n = 808$, active $n = 807$.

were observed versus the expected 91 deaths ($p < 0.001$) in the general population. It is, however, reasonable to believe that those with organ damage would have benefited at least as much as those without complications.

Main results

Compared with placebo, active treatment significantly reduced blood pressure (Figure 1). Associated with the fall in blood pressure there was a highly significant reduction in cardiovascular events. Thus, the number of primary end-points was reduced by 40% (94 versus 58; $p = 0.0031$), fatal and non-fatal stroke by 47% (53 versus 29; $p = 0.0081$), and total mortality by 43% (63 versus 36; $p = 0.0079$) (Table 3) [8]. These effects were apparent early in the study and became more pronounced with time. The reduction in total mortality was entirely due to a reduction in cardiovascular mortality (Table

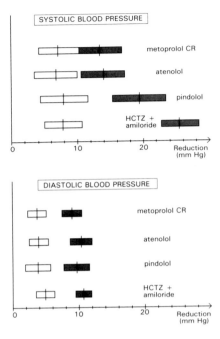

Figure 1. Supine systolic and diastolic blood pressure by treatment group and year of follow-up. Unshaded = placebo, shaded = active treatment.

3). The beneficial effects of active antihypertensive treatment were discernible at all ages studied. Of interest is also the clear effect of active treatment on the incidence of stroke in women in the present study (11.7 versus 31.1 per 1000 patient-years). In men, this effect was less impressive (25.8 versus 31.6) (Table 4) [9]. There was no difference in the attained blood pressure level between the two sexes.

During the study 172 secondary end-points occurred, 132 in the placebo group and 40 in the actively treated group ($p < 0.001$) [8]. These end-points were congestive heart failure (39 versus 19), hypertension (above 230/120 mmHg; 75 versus 10), transient ischaemic attacks (9 versus 3), and angina pectoris (9 versus 8).

Treatment and effects on blood pressure

Two months after randomization into STOP-Hypertension all patients were still on single drug therapy, and active treatment and placebo had lowered supine blood pressure by 13–25/9–11 mmHg and 7–8/4–5 mmHg, respectively (Figure 2). When comparing the "net" effects on single drug therapy,

Table 3. Primary end-points and mortality by treatment groups

	Placebo		Active		
	No	No/1000 (patient years)	No	No/1000 (patient-years)	Relative risk (94% CI)
*Primary end-points**					
All MI	28	16.5	25	14.4	0.87 (0.49, 1.56)
Fatal MI	6	3.5	6	3.5	0.98 (0.26, 3.66)
All stroke	53	31.3	29	16.8	0.53 (0.33, 0.86)
Fatal stroke	12	7.1	3	1.7	0.24 (0.04, 0.91)
Other CV death[†]	13	7.7	4	2.3	0.30 (0.07, 0.97)
Total	94	55.5	58	33.5	0.60 (0.43, 0.85)
Mortality[‡]					
Fatal MI	8	4.5	6	3.4	0.75 (0.21, 2.47)
Fatal stroke	15	8.4	4	2.3	0.27 (0.06, 0.84)
Sudden death	12	6.8	4	2.3	0.33 (0.08, 1.10)
Other CV death	6	3.4	3	1.7	0.50 (0.08, 2.34)
Total deaths**	63	35.4	36	20.2	0.57 (0.37, 0.87)

* Only the first end-point to happen.
[†] Including sudden death.
[‡] Irrespective of preceding non-fatal primary end-point.
** All causes.
MI = myocardial infarction; CV = cardiovascular; 95% CI = 95% confidence interval.

Table 4. End-point rates (number per 1000 patient-years) according to sex; relative risk (RR); 95% confidence interval (95% CI)

	Males			Females			RR Males/RR Females
	Active	Placebo	RR	Active	Placebo	RR	(95% CI)
All mortality	23.2	49.0	0.47	18.5	27.2	0.68	0.69 (0.30; 1.59)
All stroke	25.8	31.6	0.81	11.7	31.1	0.38	2.17 (0.86; 5.42)
All MI	24.2	23.7	1.02	9.0	12.2	0.73	1.39 (0.47; 4.13)

all four regimens gave approximately the same effect on diastolic blood pressure (5.3–6.4 mmHg) but HCTZ+Am was more effective in lowering systolic blood pressure (17.6 mmHg). Pindolol tended to be more effective in lowering supine systolic blood pressure (11.4 mmHg) than metoprolol CR or atenolol (6.3 and 7.2 mmHg, respectively) [10, 11]. In a separate analysis, the difference in effect on systolic blood pressure on monotherapy could not be explained by the different effects on heart rate.

After twelve months of treatment, 65% of the actively treated patients received supplementary drugs. A majority of those starting with a beta-blocker received supplementary treatment (68–78%), compared to those who started with the diuretic (40%). Approximately 80% of those receiving placebo had supplementary placebo treatment. After addition of supplementary treatment there were no significant differences in blood pressure lower-

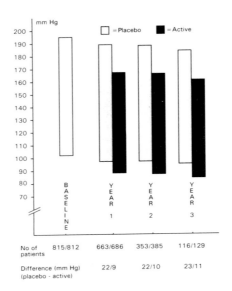

Figure 2. Reduction in systolic and diastolic blood pressure between 0 and 2 months; mean, 95% confidence intervals.

ing between the groups, which was evident already at the six-month visit. When supplementary treatment was added there was a further reduction in the blood pressure by 13.6/4.9 mmHg in the metoprolol group where 78.1% received supplementary treatment; 15.4/4.2 mmHg (68.3% supplement) in the atenolol group; 12.8/4.0 mmHg (72.5% supplement) in the pindolol group; 0.6/1.3 mmHg (40.2% supplement) in the HCTZ+Am group.

At the last follow-up before study termination in STOP-Hypertension, the supine blood pressure was 186/96 (SD 22/10) mmHg in the placebo group and 167/87 (SD 21/9) mmHg in the actively treated group (difference 19.5/8.1 mmHg). At the end of the study 77% of patients in the placebo group and 84% of those in the actively treated group were still taking the study medication and two-thirds of the actively treated patients were receiving combined treatment.

At the two-month visit the frequency of responders regarding the lowering of systolic blood pressure – defined as an achieved blood pressure below 160 mmHg or a decrease of 20 mmHg or more – was significantly higher in the group on HCTZ+Am (70%) than in those receiving a beta-blocker (33–49%) [10, 11]. After addition of supplementary treatment there were no differences in this respect between the active treatment groups (67–71%). The frequency of responders regarding the lowering of diastolic blood pressure – defined as an achieved blood pressure level below 95 mmHg or a decrease of 10 mmHg or more – was high (84–92%), and did not differ between the four active treatment regimens at either the two- or the twelve-month visit. The complete blood pressure goal in STOP-Hypertension (<160 mmHg systolic and <95 mmHg diastolic), at the two-month visit, was attained by 9–15% of the patients on beta-blockers and 30% of those receiving HCTZ+Am. At the twelve-month visit the corresponding figures had risen to 22–39% and 35%, respectively. Even so, the outcome of the STOP study was satisfactory, with a considerable reduction in the incidence of cardiovascular disease in the patients receiving active treatment.

Comparing similar patients of the same age and sex, and with the same in-study blood pressure level, the risk of stroke was significantly lower (42%, $p = 0.0402$) for patients on active therapy than for patients on placebo [12]. There was a corresponding, non-significant, reduction in cardiac events of 21%. The additional risk reduction seen with antihypertensive therapy over and above that achieved from blood pressure reduction per se was more pronounced in women than in men and decreasing with age.

We found the diastolic blood pressure to be a much stronger predictor of cardiovascular disease than the systolic blood pressure, mean arterial pressure, pulse pressure, or postural change of blood pressure [9]. We have also analysed the predictive value of systolic blood pressure alone, without the influence of diastolic blood pressure, and found the systolic blood pressure to be a very weak and non-significant predictor of cardiovascular disease.

In the whole study group ($n = 1627$) the risk of stroke increased by 3% per mmHg ($p = 0.0247$) and the risk of a cardiac event increased by 2% per mmHg ($p = 0.0376$) with increasing diastolic blood pressure for a given systolic pressure [12]. With increasing systolic blood pressure there was a non-significant decrease in stroke by 0.5% per mmHg, and a non-significant increase in cardiac event by 0.2% per mmHg for a given diastolic pressure. The cardiovascular end-points were related to the in-study diastolic blood pressure and not to the systolic one.

Metabolic and subjective side-effects

At randomization and at month 2, 6, 12, 24, 36, 48, and 60, blood was drawn with the patient in a non-fasting state and the samples were analysed at the departments of clinical chemistry at the local hospitals to which the health centres normally refer. At all visits after randomization the patients were asked about adverse effects in a structured way and if they had experienced any new symptoms since the last visit to the health centre.

No unexpected, serious, or previously unknown side-effects were evident during the study. Fifty-eight patients on active treatment and 47 on placebo discontinued randomized treatment because of subjective side-effects not classified as any specific clinical event (difference not significant).

Since the analysis was made on the intention-to-treat principle and since 23% of the patients in the placebo group were on active medication, this could be a slight underestimation of the true difference in adverse effects between the placebo and the actively treated group. However, it is obvious that active antihypertensive medication was well tolerated in this "old elderly" population.

After two months on single drug therapy a significant decrease in S-Sodium by 1.9 mmol/l in the HCTZ+Am group and an increase in S-Urate in the same group by 47 µmol/l were noted [10, 11]. After twelve months, with a majority in the beta-blocker groups on HCTZ+Am as supplementary treatment, all groups had a significant increase in both S-Urate and S-Creatinine and in all four treatment groups of the same magnitude. S-Potassium, B-Glucose, and S-Cholesterol were hardly changed at all.

The only significant differences found in the prevalence of symptoms at the two-month visit (active treatment compared with placebo in monotherapy) were more dryness in the mouth (atenolol), less swollen ankles (metoprolol CR, HCTZ+Am), more muscle discomfort/cramp (pindolol), more reduced heart rate (atenolol), and less irregular heartbeat (HCTZ+Am). At the twelve-month visit (65% with supplementary treatment) the findings were similar with a few exceptions: there were, however, no longer any differences in swollen ankles (metoprolol CR, HCTZ+Am), but there were more patients with cold hands and feet (atenolol).

Health economic aspects

A cost-effectiveness analysis has been performed and the cost-effectiveness ratio was estimated as the net cost divided by the number of life-years gained, based on hazard functions and actual costs in the trial [13]. Those ratios are low and of the same magnitude in both men and women, i.e. there is a relatively low cost per life-year gained in both sexes. However, these results cannot be extrapolated to newer drugs such as ACE-inhibitors and calcium-antagonists. Those drugs are more expensive and their ability to prevent cardiovascular disease in elderly hypertensives is unproven. Therefore a new study, STOP-Hypertension-2, has been set up in Swedish primary health care, using a novel study design, PROBE (Prospective, Randomized Open with Blinded End-point evaluation) [14], to test whether the new drugs are more cost-effective than the older ones used in STOP-Hypertension-1 [15].

In summary, the three beta-blockers and the diuretic combination used in STOP-Hypertension-1 demonstrated a highly significant reduction in fatal and non-fatal stroke and total mortality at least in the age group 70–80. Women benefited at least as much as men. This benefit was achieved in a cost-effective way with few adverse effects or metabolic disturbances.

References

1. Kannel WB, Gordon T. Evaluation of cardiovascular risk in the Framingham study. Bull NY Acad Med 1978; **54**: 573–91.
2. Collins R, Peto R, MacMahon S et al. Blood pressure, stroke, and coronary heart disease. Part 2, short-term reductions in blood pressure: overview of randomised drug trials in their epidemiological context. Lancet 1990; **335**: 827–38.
3. Coope J, Warrender TS. Randomised trial of treatment of hypertension in elderly patients in primary care. Br Med J 1986; **293**: 1145–51.
4. Amery A, Birkenhäger W, Brixko P et al. Mortality and morbidity results from the European Working Party on High Blood Pressure in the Elderly Trial (EWPHE). Lancet 1985; **i**: 1349–54.
5. Dahlöf B, Hansson L, Lindholm L, Råstam L, Scherstén B, Wester P-O. STOP-Hypertension: Swedish Trial in Old Patients with Hypertension. J Hypertens 1986; **4**: 511–3.
6. Dahlöf B, Hansson L, Lindholm L, Scherstén B, Wester P-O. STOP-Hypertension: Preliminary communication from the pilot study of the Swedish Trial in Old Patients with Hypertension. J Hypertens 1987; **5** (Suppl 5): S607–S610.
7. Hansson L, Dahlöf B, Ekbom T, Lindholm L, Scherstén B, Wester P-O. Key learnings from the STOP-Hypertension study: An update on the progress of the ongoing Swedish study of antihypertensive treatment in the elderly. Cardiovasc Drug Ther 1990; **4**: 1253–6.
8. Dahlöf B, Lindholm LH, Hansson L, Scherstén B, Ekbom T, Wester P-O. Morbidity and mortality in the Swedish Trial in Old Patients with Hypertension (STOP-Hypertension). Lancet 1991; **338**: 1281–85.
9. Ekbom T. Risks of hypertension in the elderly. Lund: Lund University, (Dissertation) 1992.
10. Ekbom T, Dahlöf B, Hansson L, Lindholm LH, Scherstén B, Wester P-O. Antihypertensive efficacy and side-effects of three beta-blockers and a diuretic in elderly hypertensives: A report from the STOP-Hypertension Study. Part 1. J Hypertens 1992; **10**: 1525–30.
11. Ekbom T, Dahlöf B, Hansson L, Lindholm LH, Scherstén B, Wester P-O. Antihypertensive efficacy and side-effects of three beta-blockers and a diuretic in elderly hypertensives: A report from the STOP-Hypertension Study, Part II. J Hypertens 1993; **11** (Suppl. 2): S19–S24.
12. Ekbom T, Dahlöf B, Hansson L, et al. The stroke preventive effect in elderly hypertensives cannot fully be explained by the reduction in office blood pressure: Insights from the Swedish Trial in Old Patients with Hypertension (STOP-Hypertension). Blood Pressure 1992; **1**: 168–72.
13. Johannesson M, Dahlöf B, Lindholm LH, et al. Treatment of hypertension in the elderly is cost-effective: An analysis of the Swedish Trial in Old Patients with Hypertension (STOP-Hypertension). J Intern Med 1993; **234**: 317–23.
14. Hansson L, Hedner T, Dahlöf B. Prospective randomized open blinded end-point (PROBE) study: A novel design for intervention trials. Blood Pressure 1992; **1**: 113–19.
15. Dahlöf B, Hansson L, Lindholm LH, et al. STOP-Hypertension 2, A prospective intervention trial of "newer" versus "older" treatment alternatives in old patients with hypertension. Blood Pressure 1993; **2**: 136–41.

7. Medical Research Council trial of treatment of hypertension in older adults: main results and treatment implications

JAMES B. CONNELLY

Introduction

In 1981 when the Medical Research Council set up their trial of the treatment of hypertension in older adults, the efficacy, safety and practicability of drug treatment for hypertension in older people was largely unknown. The existing controlled trial literature on the primary or secondary prevention of cardiovascular disease, through treatment of hypertension, was inadequate for two principal reasons. First, it had reported on only a small number of subjects and events from adults aged 60 or older at entry [1–5]. For example, the trial by Sprackling [1] involved only 60 subjects in each of the treatment and control groups, and the trial reported by Carter [2] had only 49 subjects randomised to the treatment and 48 to the control group. The second problem with the published literature in 1981 was that the larger hypertension trials, if they had considered patients aged over 60 at all, had reported these results as subgroup analyses which lacked statistical power and prompted questions rather than answered them [6–10].

The lack of information on the benefits and risks of treating older hypertensive adults was considered to be particularly unsatisfactory because, in addition to the problems already mentioned this age-group presents additional questions regarding the value of treatment. Older people are a 'survivor' group who may have taken years to 'track' to their current hypertensive status [11]. In addition, the pathophysiology of high blood pressure in older people differs from that in younger people and, it was argued, this meant that their likely response to treatment could also differ significantly from that observed in younger age-groups [9]. Moreover, it was widely believed that older patients were more prone to side-effects than younger patients [12]. In sum, it was not known whether treatment of hypertension in older adults conferred more benefits than costs.

Taking this large gap in knowledge as the starting point, the Medical

103

Gastone Leonetti and Cesare Cuspidi (eds), Hypertension in the Elderly, 103–121
© 1994 *Kluwer Academic Publishers. Printed in the Netherlands*

Research Council decided to conduct a randomised trial to compare two then current major forms of treatment with a placebo. In many countries, including the UK, the treatment of hypertension is overwhelmingly carried out at primary care level. The proposed trial, therefore, was designed to utilise a network of collaborating general practice clinics. This network had been established through the efforts of many people, in particular by William (Bill) Miall, and is now known as the MRC General Practice Research Framework (GPRF) [13].

Trial aims

The trial aimed at establishing whether antihypertensive treatment in men and women aged 65–74 years reduces mortality and morbidity due to stroke and coronary heart disease and mortality from all causes. Secondary aims were to compare the effects of the two active drugs and to see whether responses to treatment differed between men and women.

To achieve the primary aim it was estimated that 5000 men and women aged 65–74 would require follow-up for five years to allow a 30% reduction in the rate of stroke (fatal and non-fatal) to be seen between the active and placebo groups, given a power of 90% and a significance level of 2%.

Choice of systolic blood pressure as the main trial criterion

In this trial systolic rather than diastolic blood pressure was chosen as the main criterion for trial eligibility. Epidemiological studies have demonstrated that systolic blood pressure is more strongly related to the risk of occurrence of stroke than diastolic pressure [14].

The detailed methods and procedures used in the trial are described elsewhere [15], here only certain specific aspects are elaborated which may assist in the interpretation of the results. The purpose of this chapter is to describe the principal results of the MRC Older Adults trial and discuss these findings in relation to other trials and, finally, treatment recommendations.

Randomisation, target blood pressures and treatment regimens

Trial entrants were randomised in stratified blocks of eight within each sex and clinic to one of four groups: (a) a potassium sparing diuretic plus a thiazide diuretic (amiloride plus hydrochlorothiazide), or (b) a matching placebo tablet; (c) the β-blocker atenolol, or (d) a matching placebo tablet. The trial was single-blind, with patients unaware of which group they were allocated to and the doctors and nurses aware. This single-blind design was considered to be ethically necessary and ensured that general practitioners found the trial procedures acceptable.

The dosage of the diuretic combination was originally 5 mg of amiloride and 50 mg of hydrochlorothiazide; following the results of an early substudy in 1985 these dosages were altered to 2.5 mg of amiloride and 25 mg of hydrochlorothiazide in a single tablet once daily. Those randomised to the β-blocker received 50 mg of atenolol once daily.

These initial regimens were altered if necessary in order to achieve the assigned target pressure which was allocated to each subject. Each subject's target was based upon the mean level of systolic blood pressure which was measured by the trial doctor after run-in. If this mean was <180 mmHg the target was ≤150 mmHg; if it was ≥180 mmHg the target was ≤160 mmHg.

Regimens were altered in those receiving active treatment if their blood pressure had not decreased at all after 12 weeks, or if their target pressure had not been achieved after 6 months. The commonest change necessary was an increase in atenolol to 100 mg daily, occurring in 225 patients. For either active drug, supplementation, if necessary to achieve the target, was allowed by adding the other active drug. Nifedipine was then allowed, as a further supplement, in doses up to 20 mg per day given as a single dose. After this, if further supplementation was necessary, any other drug was allowed as a supplementary drug.

Follow-up

The trial entrants were followed up fortnightly for one month, then monthly up to three months, and three-monthly thereafter. At each follow up visit the research nurse measured the patient's blood pressure twice and calculated the mean. Where the mean blood pressure at any visit reached or exceeded 115 mmHg diastolic or 210 mmHg systolic, the patient was recalled a fortnight later; if either of these levels was found at that visit the management of the patient was changed. If the patient was receiving active treatment the general practitioner managed their therapy without reference to the trial drug protocol. If on placebo, the patient was transferred to active treatment; this was required in 11% of patients on placebo. Patients whose blood pressure equalled or exceeded these specified upper limits on any three non-consecutive occasions were similarly managed.

Each patient received an annual medical examination and blood was taken to measure urea, creatinine, cholesterol and electrolytes. A 12 lead ECG was obtained and, like the baseline ECG, was coded using the Minnesota code. After 12 weeks in the trial all patients filled in a self-completion questionnaire which enquired about symptoms which might be attributable to drug effects. At each follow-up visit all patients were asked to report any symptoms, compliance was stressed and a tablet count was made.

Withdrawals from randomised treatment

In addition to the blood pressure criteria for withdrawal from randomised treatment already described, other reasons for withdrawal were allowed. These included the development of complications necessitating active treatment and suspected adverse drug reactions. Patients were also allowed to be switched from placebo to active treatment if this was considered by their doctor to be clinically indicated ($n = 319$). All patients withdrawn from their randomised treatment were asked to continue to attend all follow-up visits and annual examinations, and clinics were asked to report terminating events.

Trial terminating events

Events terminating a patient's participation in the trial were: stroke, whether non-fatal or fatal; coronary events, defined as sudden death thought to be due to a coronary cause, death known to be due to a myocardial infarction, and non-fatal myocardial infarction; other cardiovascular events, including deaths due to hypertension (ICD 8th Edition 400–404) and to rupture or dissection of an aortic aneurysm; and death from any other cause. Clinic staff reported these events to the co-ordinating centre. The records of patients who suffered non-fatal terminating events and of any others who lapsed from the trial, whatever the reason, were 'flagged' at Southport NHS Central Register to ensure notification of death.

The diagnostic evidence for each terminating event was assessed by an arbitrator blind to the treatment regimen. All available documentation was reviewed, including copies of general practitioners' notes, hospital in-patient or out-patient notes, electrocardiographic recordings, necropsy findings, and death certificates. In the majority of cases the classification of fatal events used in the trial analyses was based on this detailed information rather than solely on the wording or coding of the death certificate. The arbitrator used WHO criteria [16, 17] for classification of strokes and coronary events. If a patient had a non-fatal event followed by a fatal event in the same category, only the fatal event was included in the analyses: (41 people were in this group: 19 strokes and 22 coronary events). If a person suffered two events in different categories – for example, a non-fatal stroke then a coronary event (fatal or non-fatal) then both were included: (10 people had a non-fatal stroke followed by a fatal coronary event, and 3 people had a non-fatal coronary event followed by a non-fatal stroke). Data for terminating events were analysed after every 5000 patient-years. An overall type 1 error rate of 0.02 was maintained for the main active versus placebo comparison for stroke with five analyses of the data. The comparison of event rates between the two sexes, and between the two active treatment groups was also kept under review by an independent monitoring and ethical committee.

Results

Table 1 shows the baseline characteristics of patients at trial entry and confirms that the three treatment groups were well balanced after randomis-

Table 1. Numbers entered, and characteristics of treatment groups at entry

	Men			Women		
	Diuretic	β-blocker	Placebo	Diuretic	β-blocker	Placebo
Number entered	454	456	926	627	646	1287
Mean years of observation	5.6	5.6	5.6	6.0	5.9	5.9
Mean age (years)	70.2	70.3	70.2	70.4	70.4	70.4
Mean body mass index (kg/m^2)	26.1	26.4	26.4	26.8	26.8	26.6
Mean systolic blood pressure (mmHg)	183	183	183	186	186	186
Mean diastolic blood pressure (mmHg)	92	91	91	90	91	90
Mean serum cholesterol (mmol/l)	5.9	6.0	5.9	6.9	6.9	6.8
Mean serum potassium (mmol/l)	4.2	4.2	4.2	4.2	4.2	4.2
Mean serum urate (μmol/l)	376	374	374	318	311	313
Mean serum sodium (mmol/l)	141	141	141	142	142	142
Mean serum urea (mmol/l)	6.1	6.2	6.0	5.9	5.7	5.8
% Cigarette smokers	22	21	24	14	15	13
% Ischaemic ECG*	18	17	18	17	14	15

*1_{1-3} 4_{1-3} 5_{1-2} on Minnesota code (one or more code present).

ation. The trial entered 4396 patients and the average follow-up time was 5.8 years, thus achieving 25,355 patient-years of observation.

Course of blood pressure

Based on an 'intention to treat' analysis, Figure 1 shows that both systolic and diastolic pressures fell immediately in all groups. The largest fall in systolic pressure was seen in the diuretic group during the first three months. The mean levels of systolic pressure in the two active treatment groups converged over 2 years, and thereafter were similar. The use of supplementary drugs by those randomised to β-blocker consistently exceeded that by patients randomised to the diuretic regimen; at five years 52% of the β-blocker group and 38% of the diuretic group were receiving supplementary drugs. The differential use of supplementary drugs partially explains the narrowing of the difference between these mean pressures.

In those entering the trial a difference was found between mean run-in (R) and doctor's confirmatory (E) systolic and diastolic blood pressure

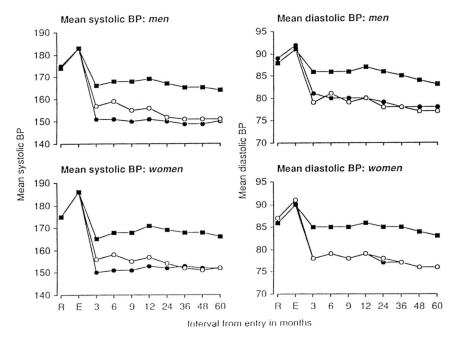

Figure 1. Mean blood pressure course by interval in trial: ■ placebo ● diuretic ○ β-blocker.

measurements. The latter being on average higher by 10 mmHg for systolic and 3mmHg for diastolic pressure.

Self-reported symptoms, withdrawals from randomised treatment and lapses from follow-up

Twelve weeks after randomisation, patients were given a questionnaire on symptoms (Table 2). Compared with those taking placebo those on the diuretic complained of significantly more faintness, numbness of the fingers or toes, pins and needles in fingers, muscle cramp and nightmares. They also reported significantly less wheeze. These symptoms did not differ between the sexes. Compared with those taking placebo, those on β-blockers complained of significantly more faintness, sleepiness, shortness of breath, diarrhoea, numbness of fingers or toes, pins and needles in the fingers and muscle cramps. The prevalence of symptoms did not differ between the sexes. A significantly higher prevalence of sleepiness, shortness of breath, wheeze and diarrhoea and a significantly lower prevalence of muscle cramp was found in the β-blocker group compared with the diuretic group. However, there was a high prevalence of many symptoms in the placebo group and even though

Table 2. Prevalence (%) of symptoms reported at 12 weeks after entry

Complaint	Both Sexes ($N = 4135$)		
	Diuretic	β-blocker	Placebo
Faintness	16.5^z	14.8^x	12.0
Faintness (standing)	57.3	49.3	52.6
Sleepy	35.8	$41.2^{a,z}$	32.5
Short of breath	24.0	$29.3^{y,b}$	23.9
Wheeze	11.0^y	15.2^b	14.4
Headaches	15.5	14.7	16.2
Diarrhoea	3.9	$8.1^{z,c}$	5.2
Vomiting	4.0	5.0	3.5
Dry eyes	6.7	7.0	6.7
Numbness	22.3^z	22.8^z	15.1
Pins & Needles	18.7^y	18.7^y	14.3
Cramp	37.2^z	$31.4^{b,x}$	27.1
Palpitations	11.3	10.4	11.3
Nightmares	11.3^x	9.9	9.1
Wakefulness	29.8	31.0	29.6

[a,b,c]Difference between diuretic and β-blocker significant at 0.05, 0.01, 0.001, respectively.
[x,y,z]Difference between diuretic and placebo or between β-blocker and placebo significant at 0.05, 0.01, 0.001, respectively.

statistically significant differences were found the absolute increases are generally small.

Table 3 shows the numbers and rates of people withdrawn from randomised treatment because of either suspected adverse reactions or blood pressure above the limits for trial. Their follow-up routine, excepting drug treatment, was the same as for those who continued to receive the randomly allocated treatment. Compared with the placebo group, the diuretic group had significantly more withdrawals for impaired glucose tolerance, gout, skin disorders, muscle cramp, nausea and dizziness. Those randomised to the β-blocker were withdrawn significantly more often compared with the placebo group for impaired glucose tolerance, Raynaud's phenomenon, dyspnoea, lethargy, nausea, dizziness, headache and low pulse rate. Those on β-blocker were withdrawn significantly more often than those on diuretic because of Raynaud's phenomenon, dyspnoea, lethargy, headache and low pulse rate and significantly less often because of gout and muscle cramps. Overall, the β-blocker group had significantly more withdrawals than the diuretic group, because of both suspected side-effects and inadequate blood pressure control.

Over the five and a half years about 25% of people were lost to follow-up. The cumulative percentages of people who stopped taking their randomised treatment, including both those withdrawn but continuing on follow-up and those lost to follow-up, were 48% of the diuretic group, 63% of the β-blocker group, and 53% of the placebo group. There were about 6300 patient-years in each of the four randomly allocated treatment groups. In the

Table 3. Principal reasons for withdrawal from randomised treatment, numbers of reports and rates/1000 patient-years

	Diuretic		β-blocker		Placebo	
	No	Rate	No	Rate	No	Rate
Impaired glucose tolerance	25	6.9[b]	17	5.8[a]	20	2.7
Gout	16	4.4[c]	0[z]	0.0[z]	1	0.1
Impotence in men	3	2.1	4	3.5	2	0.7
Raynaud's phenomenon	2	0.6	33	11.3[c,z]	2	0.3
Skin disorder	14	3.9[b]	7	2.4	8	1.1
Cramp	19	5.2[c]	3	1.0[y]	1	0.1
Dyspnoea	3	0.8	67	22.9[c,z]	8	1.1
Lethargy	15	4.1	56	19.1[c,z]	15	2.0
Nausea	27	7.4[c]	12	4.1[b]	8	1.1
Dizziness	27	7.4[c]	31	10.6[c]	9	1.2
Headache	9	2.5	21	7.2[c,y]	8	1.1
Low pulse rate	0	0.0	82	28.0[c,z]	0	0.0
Blood pressure above limit	1	0.3[c]	12	4.1[c,y]	175	23.2

[x,y,z]Difference between diuretic and β-blocker significant at 0.05, 0.01, 0.001, respectively
[a,b,c]Difference between diuretic and placebo or between β-blocker and placebo significant at 0.05, 0.01, 0.001, respectively.

diuretic group, treatment accounted for 69% of the patient years, including supplementation by the β-blocker for 11% of the time. Corresponding percentages for those allocated to the β-blocker were 55%, including supplementation with diuretic for 16%. In the placebo groups 69% of the patient years were spent on placebo treatment, with 6% of the time on either of the active treatments.

Primary results

Stroke
The number of fatal plus non-fatal strokes was significantly reduced in people randomised to receive active treatment (101 versus 134 on placebo; $p = 0.04$) giving a reduction in rates of 25% (95% CI, 3%–42%), i.e. 8.1 versus 10.8 per 1000 patient years, Table 4. There is no evidence that this effect differed in the two sexes, Table 5.

Coronary events
There were fewer events in those allocated to active treatment compared with placebo (128 versus 159; $p = 0.08$). This 19% reduction (95% CI, 2% increase to 36% reduction) was non-significant (Table 4). Coronary events were reduced in men only, but this sex difference is not significant (interaction test $p = 0.12$) (Table 5).

Table 4. Main events and rates (per 1000 patient-years) by randomised treatment group, both sexes together

Patient-years*	Diuretic 6290		β-blocker 6330		Active treatment 12620		Placebo 12735		% difference† (95% CI)	per 1000 py (95% CI)
	No	Rate	No	Rate	No	Rate	No	Rate		
Strokes										
Fatal	16	2.5	21	3.3	37	2.9	42	3.3	12 (−37–44)	0.4 (−1.0–1.8)
Non-fatal	29	4.7	35	5.6	64	5.2	92	7.4		
Total	45	7.3	56	9.0	101	8.1	134	10.8	25 (3–42)	2.7 (0.3–5.1)
Coronary events										
Fatal	33	5.2	52	8.2	85	6.7	110	8.6	22 (−4–41)	1.9 (−0.2–4.0)
Non-fatal	15	2.4	28	4.5	43	3.4	49	3.9		
Total	48	7.7	80	12.8	128	10.3	159	12.7	19 (−2–36)	2.4 (−0.2–5.0)
All cardiovascular events	107	17.4	151	24.6	258	21.0	309	25.2	17 (2–29)	4.2 (0.5–7.9)
All cardiovascular deaths	66	10.5	95	15.0	161	12.8	180	14.1	9 (−12–27)	1.3 (−1.5–4.1)
Non-cardiovascular deaths	68	10.8	72	11.4	140	11.1	135	10.6	−5 (−33–17)	−0.5 (−3.1–2.1)
Cancer deaths	49	7.8	59	9.3	108	8.6	99	7.8	−10 (−45–16)	−0.8 (−3.0–1.4)
All deaths	134	21.3	167	26.4	301	23.9	315	24.7	3 (−14–18)	0.8 (−3.0–4.6)

*Patient-years for stroke, coronary events and cardiovascular events are slightly less.
†Differences between total active group and placebo group.

Table 5. Principal events and rates (per 1000 patient-years) by sex

	Men				Women			
	Active (5075 py)*		Placebo (5192 py)*		Active (7545 py)*		Placebo (7543 py)*	
	No	Rate	No	Rate	No	Rate	No	Rate
Strokes	55	11.1	71	14.1	46	6.2	63	8.5
Coronary events	69	13.8	100	19.7	59	7.9	59	7.9
All cardiovascular events	142	29.1	182	36.9	116	15.7	127	17.3
All cardiovascular deaths	89	17.5	115	22.1	72	9.5	65	8.6
Non-cardiovascular deaths	94	18.5	65	12.5	46	6.1	70	9.3
Cancer deaths	74	14.6	47	9.1	34	4.5	52	6.9
All deaths	183	36.1	180	34.7	118	15.6	135	17.9

*Patient-years for stroke, coronary events and cardiovascular events are slightly less.

All cardiovascular events

The number of cardiovascular events was significantly reduced on active treatment (258 versus 309 placebo; $p = 0.03$) i.e. 21.0 versus 25.2 events per 1000 patient years, giving a 17% reduction (95% CI, 2–29%), Table 4. Of these events, 41% were strokes and 51% were coronary episodes. Once again, sex did not appear to influence this treatment effect, Table 5.

All-cause mortality

This was similar in the treated and placebo groups (301 versus 315 placebo) i.e. 23.9 versus 24.7 deaths per 1000 patient-years, Table 4. There was no evident sex difference in this respect (Table 5). Cardiovascular deaths were slightly fewer on active treatment (161 versus 180) but non-cardiovascular deaths were nearly equal (140 versus 135), as were cancer deaths (108 versus 99). However, cancer deaths showed a difference between the sexes: 74 active versus 47 placebo deaths in men, 34 active versus 52 placebo deaths in women (interaction test $p = 0.002$). Twenty-one of these patients had a history of cancer at trial entry (4 in the diuretic, 6 in the β-blocker and 11 in the placebo groups, respectively), their hypertension at the time being viewed as an additional and legitimate clinical concern. Omitting these cases did not alter the treatment/sex interaction ($p = 0.002$).

Subgroup results

Individual active drugs

Stroke

There were 45 strokes in the diuretic group, 56 in the β-blocker group and 134 in the placebo group (rates of 7.3, 9.0 and 10.8 per 1000 patient-years, respectively). The rates were not significantly different in the two active groups ($p = 0.33$).

Coronary events

There were 48, 80 and 159 coronary events in the diuretic, beta-blocker and placebo groups (rates of 7.7, 12.8 and 12.7 per 1000 patient-years), respectively. The rate in the diuretic group was significantly ($p = 0.006$) lower than that in the β-blocker group.

All cardiovascular events

There were 107, 151 and 309 cardiovascular events in the diuretic, β-blocker and placebo groups (rates of 17.4, 24.6, 25.2 per 1000 patient-years), respectively. The rate was significantly lower in the diuretic compared with the β-blocker group ($p = 0.007$).

All-cause mortality

The all-cause mortality difference between the diuretic and β-blocker (134 versus 167 deaths, respectively) is of marginal statistical significance ($p = 0.07$), with an observed 19% reduction (95% CI, 2% increase to 36% reduction) in the diuretic group. This difference is due to cardiovascular deaths (66 diuretic versus 95 β-blocker; $p = 0.03$) there being similar numbers of non-cardiovascular deaths (68 diuretic versus 72 β-blocker). The main category of non-cardiovascular death was cancer. The apparent male excess of cancer deaths is somewhat more pronounced on β-blocker than on diuretic (43 versus 31, $p = 0.19$). Comparing β-blocker with placebo, there is a marked sex/treatment interaction ($p = 0.002$): in men, cancer death rates are 17.0 and 9.1 per 1000 patient-years, respectively, while in women rates are 4.2 and 6.9 per 1000 patient-years, respectively. As previously, exclusion of cancers at entry did not substantially alter the sex/treatment interaction ($p = 0.002$). Classification of the cancer deaths by site and randomised treatment group showed no organ or system clustering, except that men randomised to β-blocker showed 14 cancers of the lung or bronchus compared to 8 and 11 in the diuretic and placebo groups, giving rates per 1000 patient-years of 5.5, 3.1 and 2.1, respectively.

Cigarette smoking

Effect of active treatment

For every end-point the event rates were raised in smokers compared with non-smokers, and there is some evidence that smokers and non-smokers differed in their response to active treatment with respect to stroke events and all cardiovascular events (interaction tests, $p = 0.04$ and 0.03, respectively). In both cases the reduction in events on active treatment appeared to be confined to non-smokers, and this was so for both men and women. However, for coronary events and all-cause mortality there was no evidence

Table 6. Principal events by entry smoking habit and randomly allocated drug, both sexes together

	Smokers				Non-smokers			
	Diuretic	β-blocker	Total active	Placebo	Diuretic	β-blocker	Total active	Placebo
Patient years*	1298	1300	2598	2707	4985	5030	10015	10023
	No	No	No	No	No	No	No	No
	(Rate)	(Rate)	(Rate)	(Rate)	(Rate)	(Rate)	(Rate)	(Rate)
Strokes	17	17	34	29	28	39	67	105
	(13.5)	(13.5)	(13.5)	(10.9)	(5.7)	(7.9)	(6.8)	(10.7)
Coronary	13	28	41	46	35	52	87	113
events	(10.1)	(21.9)	(16.0)	(17.4)	(7.1)	(10.5)	(8.8)	(11.4)
All	37	55	92	84	70	96	166	225
cardiovascular	(29.6)	(44.4)	(37.0)	(32.2)	(14.3)	(19.6)	(17.0)	(23.3)
events								
Non-	17	28	45	37	51	44	95	98
cardiovascular	(13.1)	(21.5)	(17.3)	(13.7)	(10.2)	(8.8)	(9.5)	(9.8)
deaths								
All deaths	39	68	107	98	95	99	194	217
	(30.0)	(52.3)	(41.2)	(36.2)	(19.1)	(19.7)	(19.4)	(21.6)

*Patient-years for stroke, coronary events and cardiovascular events are slightly less.

that response to active treatment differed between smokers and non-smokers. When compared with diuretic, the response to β-blocker was significantly modified by smoking status for all cause mortality ($p = 0.04$), there being no suggestion of an interaction for cause-specific end-points.

Entry systolic blood pressure (160–179 mmHg and 180–209 mmHg), diastolic blood pressure (<90 mmHg or ≥90 mmHg), and age (65–69 or 70–74)

There was no evidence that these characteristics had any influence on treatment responses. This applies equally to the average of the three run-in blood pressures and the doctors' confirmatory pressures.

On treatment analyses

All results so far have been on the 'intention-to-treat' principle. This approach though unbiased has the disadvantage that possible drug effects might be diluted by the substantial proportion of patient-years which did not follow the assigned treatment.

An additional analysis was therefore carried out for cardiovascular deaths and for cancer deaths in relation to actual treatment received. For cardiovascular events, deaths rather than non-fatal events are examined since the latter would be less reliably reported once patients had been lost to follow-up. However, this analysis should be viewed as secondary since one cannot correct for the fact that changes in treatment may be related to the patient's risk of death. The on-treatment results include only those deaths and patient-years on randomised treatment. For diuretic and β-blocker groups this includes any periods spent either with altered dose of their randomised drug or whilst taking the randomised drug in combination with other drugs (including β-blocker or diuretic, respectively). Cardiovascular deaths were 28, 40 and 87 (giving rates per 1000 patient-years of 6.5, 11.5 and 9.9 in the diuretic, β-blocker and placebo groups, respectively). Cancer deaths were 12, 22, 19 in men (giving rates of 6.9, 15.8 and 5.3 per 1000 patient-years in the diuretic, β-blocker and placebo groups, respectively); and 8, 6, 32, in women (giving rates of 3.1, 2.9, 6.2 per 1000 patient-years in the diuretic, β-blocker and placebo groups, respectively) [15].

The on-treatment death rates for cardiovascular and cancer deaths are lower than the corresponding 'intention-to-treat' rates, since death rates were higher after patients had withdrawn from randomised trial therapy or had lapsed from follow-up. However, the differences in cardiovascular and cancer death rates "on-treatment" follow the same pattern as described by the "intention-to-treat" approach.

Logistic regression analyses

Logistic regression analyses have been used to relate randomised treatment to the risk of subsequent major events after controlling for possible confounding factors, Figure 2. There was no evidence of a treatment/sex interaction for any of the primary end-points.

Stroke
The beneficial effect of diuretic compared with placebo is estimated as a statistically significant 31% reduction (95% CI, 3%–51%) in risk, after allowance for baseline factors. The reduction in the β-blocker group was not statistically significant.

Coronary heart disease
There is a highly significant estimated 44% reduction (95% CI, 21%–60%) in risk in the diuretic group compared with placebo after allowance for baseline factors. The β-blocker group shows no difference from the placebo group. There was no evidence of an effect modification on these results in those with abnormal base-line ECG findings.

All cardiovascular events and cardiovascular deaths
The diuretic group showed a marked reduction in risk, (35% and 29%; 95% CI, 17%–49% and 4%–48%, respectively) after allowance for baseline factors whereas the β-blocker group did not.

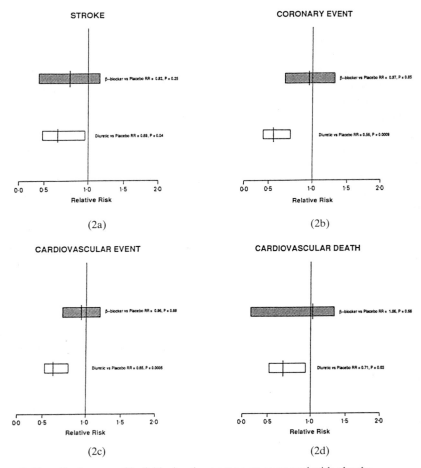

Figure 2. The effectiveness of individual active treatments compared with placebo.

Total deaths
The key predictors were: sex, age, smoking and ischaemic changes on ECG. Concerning cholesterol, a non-significant inverse association is observed, which suggests that low cholesterol may be associated with an increased risk of non-cardiovascular deaths. Because diuretic treatment was not associated with a reduction in non-cardiovascular deaths the 16% observed reduction (93% CI, 5% increase to 33% reduction) in total mortality was not significant.

Discussion

The overall results of this trial show that active treatment led to a significant reduction in cardiovascular events in men and women aged 65–74 with sustained mild to moderate levels of hypertension. The observed differences between the primary active drugs in preventing cardiovascular morbidity and mortality stem primarily from the apparent effectiveness of the diuretic in reducing coronary events and deaths. This interesting finding is contrary to expectations relating to the potential adverse metabolic effects of diuretics, particularly a rise in low-density lipoprotein and therefore total cholesterol. However, the increases in total cholesterol, averaged over the period from 3 months after entry to the end of follow-up, were identical and small (0.1 mmol/l) in all three randomised groups. A larger increase occurred in the serum urate levels on active treatment ([entry/in trial mean] 343/388; 337/372; 338/342 μmol/l for diuretic, β-blocker and placebo, respectively) but evidently these did not prevent the beneficial effect of the diuretic on cardiovascular events. Those in the diuretic group experienced a more rapid and greater control of their blood pressure compared to the β-blocker group (Figure 1) and this may have contributed to the differences in effectiveness with regard to coronary events.

All-cause mortality was not significantly affected by active treatment (Table 4). However, cancer death rates were apparently increased in men but not in women randomised to active treatment, and when individual active treatments were compared to placebo, men but not women randomised to the β-blocker had significantly increased cancer death rates. No explanation for this finding can be given; it should be remembered, however, that cancer was not a primary end-point in this trial, and the finding is subject to all the uncertainties of post hoc and sub-group analysis. Furthermore, diagnoses of cancer were not adjudicated in the same formal way as were the primary trial end-points. The results may be a chance finding which would need more substantial evidence to justify further action. Indeed, since the publication of these results two studies [18, 19] have found no evidence of any association between β-blockers and cancer.

An overview of fourteen randomised trials of antihypertensive treatment, combining trials using different active drugs and different age-ranges, reported a statistically significant average 14% reduction in coronary heart disease events in those receiving active treatment [20]. However, this trial, like other individual trials [21–23], has demonstrated no primary cardioprotective effect of β-blockade, even though the effectiveness of acute and long-term β-blockade in reducing mortality after myocardial infarction has been amply demonstrated [24–28]. This lack of a distinct primary cardioprotective effect of β-selective β-blockers, when directly compared to a diuretic regimen, has previously been reported in middle-aged men in the Heart Attack Primary Prevention in Hypertension (HAPPHY) trial [23]. The procedures of the HAPPHY trial ensured that both the β-blocker and diuretic groups

attained equal reductions in diastolic blood pressure. The lack of a cardioprotective effect of the β-blocker in the present trial may, therefore, have been
due to the greater systolic blood pressure lowering in the diuretic group. To
examine this a logistic regression model of in-trial risk factor values was
fitted for cardiovascular events, the treatment term comparing the diuretic
with the β-blocker. This procedure therefore allowed for a statistical adjust-
ment of in-trial effects, so that treatment effects given equivalent reductions
in blood pressure could be studied. This demonstrated that even adjusting
for blood pressure changes, the diuretic was associated with a lower risk of
cardiovascular events ($p = 0.01$) compared with the β-blocker. This opens
up an interesting speculation that the active treatments differed in their
effects on a third factor, or factors, which influenced outcome. These results
add to this possibility, which was first raised by the findings of the earlier
MRC trial in middle-aged people [21].

Whilst the present trial was in progress four randomised controlled trials
of antihypertensive drug therapy in men and women aged 60 and over were
reported [29–32]. In the European Working Party on High Blood Pressure
in the Elderly (EWPHE) trial [29] there were comparable and significant
reductions in cardiac and cardiovascular deaths and a non-significant reduction in fatal stroke.

The trial by Coope and Warrender of treatment of hypertension in elderly
patients in primary care [30] recruited 884 hypertensive patients (30% men)
aged 60 to 79 years in 13 general practices and followed them for 4.4 years.
Active treatment was started with atenolol 100 mg daily and was then supple-
mented with bendrofluazide 5 mg daily, if necessary. The combined regime
accounted for most of the active treatment in this trial, followed by atenolol
on its own. The results showed a beneficial effect of treatment on stroke.
Coronary events, unlike in the present trial, were not affected. An excess of
cancers amongst those on active treatment was not significant and was described as 'fortuitous'.

The Swedish trial in old patients (STOP) [31] reported significant relative
risk reductions for stroke, fatal stroke and all-cause mortality of 47%, 76%
and 43%, respectively. The proportions initially allocated to the β-blockers
(metoprolol, pindolol, atenolol) and the diuretic combination (amiloride plus
hydrochlorothiazide) were not given in the published results [31], however,
two-thirds of the actively treated group received the diuretics in addition to
a β-blocker [31].

The sub-group analyses in smokers and non-smokers are post hoc and
therefore cautious interpretation is required [33]. Strokes and all cardiovascular events were prevented by active treatment only in non-smokers. In the
present trial, like the earlier MRC trial [13], blood pressure control in
smokers was poorer, especially in the β-blocker groups (atenolol and popranolol, respectively).

A large proportion (43%) of randomised participants had a systolic pressure equal to or exceeding 160 mmHg and a diastolic pressure below 90

mmHg (thus meeting the definition for Isolated Systolic Hypertension). There was no evidence that the overall trial results were not applicable to this subgroup. This conclusion is supported by the Systolic Hypertension in the Elderly Programme (SHEP) which showed a significant 37% reduction in stroke risk amongst men and women randomised to a stepped care regimen (chlorthalidone step 1, atenolol step 2) compared to a placebo group [32]. Myocardial infarction and cardiovascular events (which included coronary bypass grafting and angioplasty) in the active treatment group compared with placebo were reduced by 33% and 32%, respectively. The SHEP trial did not report any excess in cancer deaths in the active treatment group.

The present trial differs from the earlier MRC trial of treatment of mild hypertension in middle-aged adults [13, 21] in showing the effectiveness of the diuretic in reducing coronary events. The explanation of this difference may derive from the differences in the diuretics used or in the nature of hypertension and responses to treatment with age, and these possibilities are not mutually exclusive.

The clinical decision to use drugs to treat asymptomatic older people who have levels of sustained hypertension in the range considered here should be informed by the effectiveness of the treatment policy, the absolute and relative risks for the individual patient due to the profile of risk-factors they carry, the adverse drug reactions, and the non-pharmacological alternatives. Based on absolute risk reductions, the results of the present trial may be used to calculate the numbers to be treated for 5 years to avoid one event. This number decreases as the number of risk factors carried by the individual increases [15], and this illustrates the importance of considering the cardiovascular risk profile and not simply the level of hypertension presented by patients. This insight, along with the fundamental requirement that treatment decisions be based on the findings regarding efficacy and effectiveness derived from controlled trial results, has informed recent statements of treatment guidance [34, 35]. With regard to all-cause mortality, this trial, in common with others of similar size [20], did not have sufficient power to detect small effects of treatment. In addition, the complex question of whether there are patients in whom lowering blood pressure too much actually increases risk, the so-called J-shaped curve phenomenon [36–38], has not been addressed in this trial. Though results from a meta-analysis of trials [20] does not support the existence of this phenomenon, a specifically designed controlled trial is the appropriate means of deciding this issue.

Overall, then, the results suggest that treatment of hypertension using the diuretic combination reduces the risk of strokes and all cardiovascular events, at least in non-smokers. Furthermore, there is strong evidence that in this age group the diuretic combination but not the β-blocker confers considerable benefits by reducing coronary event rates.

Acknowledgements

I would like to thank the Chairman of the MRC Working Party, Professor Sir Stanley Peart, and Professor T.W. Meade for their advice and comments on this chapter.

References

1. Sprackling ME, Mitchell JRA, Short AH, Watt G. Blood pressure reduction in the elderly: A randomised controlled trial of methyldopa. Br Med J 1981; **283**: 1151–3.
2. Carter AB. Hypotensive therapy in stroke survivors. Lancet 1970; **i**: 485–9.
3. Kuramoto K, Matsushita S, Kuwajima I, Murakami M. Prospective study on the treatment of mild hypertension in the aged. Jap Heart J 1981; **22**: 75–85.
4. Morgan TO, Adams WR, Hodgson M, Gibberd RW. Failure of therapy to improve prognosis in elderly males with hypertension. Med J Aust 1980; **ii**: 27–31.
5. Hypertension – Stroke Co-operative Study Group. Effect of anti-hypertensive treatment on stroke recurrence. JAMA 1974; **229**: 409–18.
6. Veterans Administration Co-operative Study on Antihypertensive Agents. Effect of treatment on morbidity in hypertension: Results in patients with diastolic blood pressure averaging 115 through 129 mmHg. JAMA 1967; **202**: 1028–34.
7. Veterans Administration Co-operative Study Group on Antihypertensive Agents. Effects of treatment on morbidity in hypertension II: Results in patients with diastolic blood pressure averaging 90 through 114 mmHg. JAMA 1970; **213**: 1143–52.
8. Veterans Administration Co-operative Study Group on Antihypertensive Agents. Effects of treatment on morbidity in hypertension III: Influence of age, diastolic pressure and prior cardiovascular disease. Circulation 1972; **45**: 991–1004.
9. Management Committee. Treatment of mild hypertension in the elderly: A study initiated and administered by the National Heart Foundation of Australia. Med J Aust 1981; **2**: 398–402.
10. Hypertension Detection and Follow-up Program Co-operative Group. Five-year findings of the Hypertension Detection and Follow-up Programme II: Mortality by race, sex and age. JAMA 1979; **242**: 2572–6.
11. Beard K, Bulpitt C, Mascie-Taylor H et al. Management of elderly patients with sustained hypertension. Br Med J 1992; **304**: 412–6.
12. The Working Group on Hypertension in the Elderly. Statement on Hypertension in the Elderly. JAMA 1986; **256**: 70–4.
13. Miall WE, Greenburg G. Mild Hypertension: is there pressure to treat? Cambridge: Cambridge University Press 1987.
14. Kannel WB, Wolf PA, McGee DL et al. Systolic blood pressure, arterial rigidity, and risk of stroke. The Framingham Study. JAMA 1981; **245**: 1225–9.
15. Medical Research Council Working Party. MRC trial of treatment of hypertension in older adults: Principal results. Br Med J 1992; **304**: 405–12.
16. Aho H, Harmsen P, Hatano S, Marquardsen W, Smirnov VE, Strasser T. Cerebrovascular disease in the community: Results of a WHO collaborative study. Bull WHO 1980; **58**: 113–30.
17. World Health Organisation Regional Office for Europe. Myocardial infarction community register. Copenhagen: WHO 1976 (Public Health in Europe No. 5).
18. Hole DJ, Hawthorne VM, Isles CG et al. Incidence and mortality from cancer in hypertensive patients. Br Med J 1993; **306**: 609–11.
19. Fletcher AE, Beevers DG, Bulpitt CJ et al. Cancer mortality and atenolol treatment. Br Med J 1993; **306**: 622–3.

20. Collins R, Peto R, MacMahon S et al. Blood pressure, stroke, and coronary heart disease. Part 2, short-term reduction in blood pressure: Overview of randomised drug trials in their epidemiological context. Lancet 1990; **335**: 827–38.

21. Medical Research Council Working Party. MRC trial of treatment of mild hypertension: Principal results. Br Med J 1985; **291**: 97–104.

22. IPPPSH Collaborative Group: Cardiovascular Risk and Risk Factors in a Randomised Trial of Treatment Based on the Beta-blocker Oxprenolol: The International Prospective Primary Prevention Study in Hypertension (IPPPSH). J. Hypertens 1985; **3**: 379–92.

23. Wilhelmsen L, Berglund G, Elmfeldt D, et al. Beta-blockers versus diuretics in hypertensive men: Main results from the HAPPHY trial. J. Hyperten 1987; **5**: 561–72.

24. Beta-blocker Heart Attack Trial Research Group. A randomised trial of popranolol in patients with acute myocardial infarction: I. Mortality results. JAMA 1982; **247**: 1707–14.

25. Brown MA, Norris RM, Barnaby PF, Geary GG, Brandt PW. Effect of early treatment with popranolol on left ventricular function four weeks after myocardial infarction. Br Heart J 1985; **54**: 351–6.

26. MIAMI Trial Research Group. Metoprolol in acute myocardial infarction (MIAMI): A randomised placebo-controlled trial. Eur Heart J 1985; **6**: 199–226.

27. ISIS-I (First International Study of Infarct Survival) Collaborative Group. Randomised trial of intravenous atenolol among 16,027 cases of suspected acute myocardial infarction: ISIS-I. Lancet 1986; **2**: 57–66.

28. Intravenous beta-blockade during acute myocardial infarction (Editorial). Lancet 1986; **2**: 79–80.

29. Amery A, Birkenhager W, Brixko P et al. Mortality and morbidity results from the European Working Party on High Blood Pressure in the Elderly trial. Lancet 1985; **1**: 1349–54.

30. Coope J, Warrender TS. Randomised trial of treatment of hypertension in the elderly in primary care. Br Med J 1986; **293**: 1145–51.

31. Dahlöf B, Lindholm LH, Hansen L et al. Morbidity and mortality in the Swedish trial in old patients with hypertension (STOP-Hypertension). Lancet 1991; **338**: 1281–5.

32. SHEP Co-operative Research Group. Prevention of stroke by antihypertensive drug treatment in older persons with isolated systolic hypertension: Final results of the systolic hypertension in the elderly program (SHEP). JAMA 1991; **265**: 3255–64.

33. Pocock SJ, Hugher MD, Lee RJ. Statistical problems in the reporting of clinical trials. N Engl J Med 1987; **317**: 426–32.

34. Jackson R, Barham P, Bills J, et al. Management of raised blood pressure in New Zealand: A discussion document. Br Med J 1993; **307**: 107–10.

35. Sever P, Beevers G, Bulpitt C et al. Management guidelines in essential hypertension: Report of the second working party of the British Hypertension Society. Br Med J 1993; **306**: 93–7.

36. Cruickshank JM, Thorp JP, Zacharias FJ. Benefits and potential harm of lowering high blood pressure. Lancet 1987; **1**: 581–4.

37. Staessen J, Bulpitt C, Clement D, et al. Relation between mortality and treated blood pressure in elderly patients with hypertension: Report of the European Working Party on High Blood Pressure in the Elderly. Br Med J 1989; **298**: 1552–6.

38. Samuelsson OG, Wilhelmsen LW, Pennert KM, Wedel H, Berglund GL. The J-shaped relationship between coronary heart disease and achieved blood pressure level in treated hypertension; further analyses of twelve years of follow up of treated hypertensives in the Primary Prevention Trial in Gothenburg, Sweden. J. Hypertens 1990; **8**: 547–55.

8. The systolic hypertension in the elderly program*

H. MITCHELL PERRY, Jr., KENNETH G. BERGE, M. DONALD
BLAUFOX, BARRY R. DAVIS, RICHARD H. GRIMM,
ROBERT McDONALD, SARA PRESSEL, ELEANOR SCHRON,
W. McFATE SMITH, and THOMAS M. VOGT

Introduction

The Systolic Hypertension in the Elderly Program (SHEP) was a randomized
multicenter double-blind placebo-controlled trial designed to test the efficacy
of antihypertensive drug treatment in persons 60 years of age or older who
had isolated systolic hypertension (ISH). ISH was defined as a systolic blood
pressure (SBP) (160–219 mmHg) and a diastolic blood pressure (DBP)
(< 90 mmHg). Prior to the completion of SHEP, ISH remained the most
important unresolved therapeutic problem involving hypertension; no defini-
tive data were available on the possible benefits of treating this condition.
Previous randomized controlled trials on efficacy of antihypertensive drug
treatment, including the few that included older people in their samples,
have focused primarily on the problem of elevated DBP (90 mmHg or higher)
and used diastolic hypertension as the sole or main entry criterion.

   Population studies have shown that ISH is associated with increased risk
of stroke, coronary heart disease, all cardiovascular disease and all-cause
mortality in the elderly. ISH in the elderly is characterized by loss of arterial
compliance. It is rare among patients less than 50 years of age, but its
prevalence rises progressively and markedly with age, particularly after age
60, in both men and women, blacks and whites. When SHEP was planned,
it was estimated that there were more than 3 000 000 people over age 60 in
the United States with ISH. The magnitude of the problem, coupled with
the lack of knowledge on efficacy and safety of drug treatment of ISH, was
the major stimulus for the SHEP trial.

Gastone Leonetti and Cesare Cuspidi (eds), Hypertension in the Elderly, 123–137
© 1994 *Kluwer Academic Publishers. Printed in the Netherlands*

Objectives

The primary objective of the SHEP was to determine whether the long-term administration of antihypertensive drug therapy for the treatment of isolated systolic hypertension (ISH) in elderly persons reduces the combined incidence of fatal and non-fatal stroke.

Secondary objectives of SHEP included evaluations of:

1. The effect of long-term antihypertensive therapy on cardiovascular morbidity and mortality in elderly people with ISH,
2. The effect of long-term antihypertensive therapy on other selected morbidity and on mortality from any cause in elderly people with ISH,
3. Possible adverse effects of chronic use of antihypertensive drug treatment in this population,
4. The effect of therapy on indices of quality of life,
5. The natural history of ISH in the placebo population.

Two major prior subgroup hypotheses formulated for analysis were:

1. Treatment of ISH will reduce incidence of total stroke to a greater degree in those not already receiving antihypertensive medication than in those with prior treatment,
2. Treatment of ISH will reduce incidence of all myocardial events, including sudden and rapid cardiac death, in those with resting ECG abnormalities at baseline to a lesser degree than in those with normal baseline ECG's.

SHEP pilot study

SHEP was preceded by a pilot study (SHEP-PS). At the time the SHEP-PS was undertaken there was very little information about the efficacy of antihypertensive drugs in lowering SBP of elderly persons, and it was unknown whether such drugs might have negative cognitive, mood, and other side-effects unique to ISH in the elderly. It was also unclear as to whether dose regimens derived from studies of younger persons were appropriate for the elderly. The major objectives of SHEP-PS were to test the feasibility of recruitment and the efficacy and acceptability of the treatment regimen. Treatment with diuretic, plus a second antihypertensive agent if needed, was compared to treatment with placebo. Patients were randomized in a 4/1 ratio of active/placebo medication so that it would be possible to test for several second step agents. An additional six months of intervention was conducted at the end of the SHEP-PS in order to determine the efficacy of reduced doses of chlorthalidone and beta-blocker (metoprolol) in maintaining blood pressure control. This extension was sufficiently successful that reduced doses were used in the full SHEP trial.

SHEP-PS was a double-blind placebo-controlled trial which randomized

551 participants 60 years of age or older with ISH and followed them for an average of 34 months. The populations of SHEP-PS and SHEP were similar with respect to age, sex, racial distribution, and percentage under treatment at initial contact. However, the mean baseline SBP in the pilot study was about 2 mmHg higher than in SHEP; moreover, 25% of SHEP-PS participants had baseline SBP's above 180 mmHg versus 15% of SHEP participants.

Although chlorthalidone was the first step agent in both studies, the original doses in SHEP-PS were twice the doses used in the full scale study. Of 408 SHEP-PS participants on study medications at the end of the trial, only 13% of those randomized to active drugs were taking any step 2 medications; whereas 57% of the placebo participants were taking step 2 medication. Thus, 87% of patients with ISH were adequately controlled by 50 mg or less of chlorthalidone.

Although the number of events in SHEP-PS was too small to demonstrate a significant difference between the event rates in the active and placebo groups, the stroke rates in the pilot study were very similar to those in SHEP. The incidence rates for all strokes were 9.0 and 10.2 events per 1000 drug treated participants per year in SHEP-PS and SHEP, respectively. In the placebo treated participants, the comparable rates were 16.4 and 19.2. In SHEP-PS these rates included *possible* as well as *definite* strokes; if the possible strokes were excluded the stroke rates of SHEP-PS decreased to 8.3 and 12.8 for active drug and placebo participants, respectively.

SHEP-PS demonstrated the feasibility of recruitment, although 75,000 individuals had to be contacted in order to enroll 551. It also demonstrated the efficacy and acceptability of the treatment regimen.

The SHEP study

Methods

Design
SHEP was designed to determine if antihypertensive drug treatment could lower the incidence of fatal plus non-fatal stroke. It was estimated that a sample size of 4800 participants was adequate to detect a reduction in total stroke incidence of at least 32% with 90% power and a two-sided α of 0.05 after allowing for dropouts (16%) and cross-overs (19%).

Administrative organization
The participating units of the trial were a Coordinating Center, 16 Clinical Centers, an ECG Laboratory, a Central Laboratory, a CT Scan Reading Center, a Drug Distribution Center, and a Project Office. A Steering Committee, composed of a chairman, the SHEP Principal Investigators (one from each of the clinical centers) and NHLBI and NIA staff, was the decision-

making body for the scientific and technical conduct of the study. There was also an independent Data and Safety Monitoring Board.

Recruitment and screening

Mass mailing and community screening were the primary recruiting techniques. All blood pressures were measured by trained and certified technicians using standardized techniques with a standard manometer at the initial contact and a Hawksley random-zero manometer at baseline and all follow-up visits. The SBP was defined as the pressure at the first Korotkoff sound, and the DBP as the pressure at the last Korotkoff sound.

At the initial contact, those persons with a pacemaker, a recent M.I. or coronary bypass, current use of anticoagulants, stroke residual, and those considered unlikely to complete the trial because of plans to move, illness or noncompliance were excluded. In addition, individuals were excluded if they were less than 60 years old or had seated SBPs below 150 mmHg if untreated or below 130 mmHg if treated. For persons not receiving antihypertensive drugs, two additional readings were taken. When the mean of the last two readings was between 160 and 219 mmHg for SBP and less than 100 mmHg for DBP, that person was eligible for the first baseline visit.

With the agreement of patient and physician, persons receiving antihypertensive medication who had SBP's between 130 and 219 mmHg and DBP's less than 85 mmHg had their drugs withdrawn during multiple drug evaluation visits over a 2- to 8-week period in order to determine blood pressure eligibility off medication. Once off medication, they had to meet the same criteria as previously untreated persons.

The baseline phase of the trial consisted of two visits. When the average of four seated blood pressure measurements, two at each of these visits, was between 160 and 219 mmHg for SBP and less than 90 mmHg for DBP that person was blood pressure eligible. Persons were excluded on the basis of history and/or signs of major cardiovascular disease or other major disease, e.g., cancer, alcoholic liver disease, or renal dysfunction. Screenees also underwent a physical examination and behavioral assessment (including cognition, mood, and activities of daily living). A 12-lead ECG was done with a 2-minute rhythm strip, and blood was drawn.

Randomization

The coordinating center randomized participants to either active medication or matched placebo, stratifying by clinical center and by antihypertensive medication status at initial contact. The clinical centers were blinded as to a participant's group.

Treatment program

The choice of drugs in SHEP was based on objective data from previous studies. The data supporting the efficacy and safety of chlorthalidone and atenolol were strong and clear. Such was not the case for the newer more expensive ACE inhibitors and calcium-entry blockers. Moreover, SHEP-PS, which specifically dealt with isolated systolic hypertension for the first time, found that chlorthalidone alone was sufficiently effective in controlling this type of hypertension that a second drug was rarely needed.

For participants with baseline SBP greater than 180 mmHg, the goal of treatment was a reduction to less than 160 mmHg. For those with SBP's in the 160–179 mmHg range, the goal was a reduction of at least 20 mmHg. The objective of the stepped-care treatment program was to maintain SBP at or below the goal with minimum drug. All participants were initially given 12.5 mg of chlorthalidone (step 1 drug) per day or matching placebo. In an effort to reach goal blood pressure, the dose of the step 1 drug could be doubled, a step 2 drug added and then doubled in a stepwise manner unless intolerable side effects or potentially serious changes in blood chemistry (collectively termed adverse effects) occurred. A beta-blocker (atenolol) (25 mg/d) was the usual second-step drug. When it was contraindicated, reserpine (0.05 mg/d) was substituted. Potassium supplements were given to participants who had serum potassium levels below 3.2 mmol/l at any visit. Those between 3.2–3.5 mmol/l needed confirmation of that level on a second sample before supplements were given.

Blood pressure follow-up procedures
Participants were followed monthly until goal or the maximum tolerable level of stepped-care treatment was reached. All participants had quarterly visits at which blood pressure, heart rate, and body weight were recorded. An interval medical history and review of medication was obtained. At semiannual visits, standardized questionnaires were administered to screen for depression and cognitive impairment. Annual visits also included a detailed medical history, a complete physical examination, laboratory tests, and assessment of activities of daily life. An ECG was also done at the second and final annual visits. Other visits were scheduled as needed, and in particular if the blood pressure rose above escape criteria despite maximal protocol therapy. Escape criteria included: (1) SBP greater than 240 mmHg or DBP greater than 115 mmHg at a single visit, or (2) sustained SBP greater than 220 mmHg or sustained DBP greater than 90 mmHg. This was an indication to use known active drugs. When drug related adverse conditions occurred, study medication could be reduced or discontinued. If possible, therapy was resumed when it appeared safe, when the participant's blood pressure was above goal, and when the participant agreed.

Ascertainment of end-points
Stroke, the primary endpoint, was defined as rapid onset of a new neurologic deficit attributed to obstruction or rupture in the arterial system which had persisted for at least 24 hours (unless death supervened) and had to include specific localizing findings confirmed by neurologic examination or brain scan without evidence of an underlying nonvascular cause.

Definitions of the most important secondary end points were: (1) myocardial infarction – typical symptoms consistent with acute myocardial infarction plus ECG changes or significant enzyme elevation (1.25 times normal), but not including silent myocardial infarction. Fatal myocardial infarction required autopsy or death certificate diagnosis plus preterminal hospitalization with a definite or suspected diagnosis of myocardial infarction within 4 weeks of death; (2) sudden and rapid cardiac death – death within 24 hours of the onset of severe cardiac symptoms and unrelated to other known causes; (3) left ventricular failure – at least one typical symptom, such as significant dyspnea plus a chest roentgenogram characteristic of congestive heart failure or an abnormal physical sign, such as rales or ankle edema; (4) transient ischemic attack – rapid onset of a focal neurologic deficit lasting more than 30 seconds and less than 24 hours.

Decisions on occurrence of study events were made by a coding panel of three physicians blind to randomization allocation. For neurologic events the panel included two neurologists, and for cardiovascular events it included two cardiologists. Adverse clinical effects were evaluated by laboratory tests or by a standardized questionnaire asking about side effects at annual visits or when complaints were thought to be due to SHEP medication.

The assessment of cognition and mood included a questionnaire administered at baseline and semiannually. Specified questionnaire scores called for expert diagnostic evaluation by a SHEP neurologist. A diagnosis of dementia made by such an evaluation had to be confirmed by the SHEP coding panel; diagnoses of depression were not reviewed centrally, but were confirmed when possible by a psychologist/psychiatrist at the clinical centers.

Results

Recruitment

Recruitment was carried out at 16 clinical centers between 1 March 1985 and 15 January 1988. A total of 447 921 individuals aged 60 years and above were screened, and 4736 of them were randomized into the trial.

Screenees meeting blood pressure criteria and not receiving antihypertensive medication had two baseline visits. A total of 3161 such participants were randomized. Screenees taking medication and meeting blood pressure criteria for that group underwent drug withdrawals before their two baseline visits. A total of 1575 such participants were randomized. The yield from initial contact to randomization for those not taking antihypertensive medications was 1.24% and for those taking medication was 0.82%. Of those who were ineligible, 90% were excluded because of failure to meet blood pressure criteria.

Baseline characteristics

Mean age of participants was 72 years, 57% were women, and 14% were black. Forty-two percent were in their 60's, 45% in their 70's, and 14% were

80 years of age or older. Mean SBP at baseline was 170.3 mmHg; mean DBP was 76.6 mmHg. For 57% of participants, baseline SBP was 160–169 mmHg; for 27% it was 170–179 mmHg; for 10% it was 180–189 mmHg; and for 5% it was 190 mmHg or more. Of all participants, 1.4% reported a history of stroke, and 5% reported a history of myocardial infarction. On physical examination, 7% had carotid bruits. ECG abnormality was present at baseline in 61%. As a group, the cohort was overweight, with a body-mass index averaging 27.5 kg/m^2 (almost 30% overweight by actuarial criteria). Fewer than 1% had evidence of cognitive impairment, and 11% manifested symptoms of depression based on standardized questionnaire criteria. Only 5% reported limitation in activities of daily living.

Adherence to protocol drugs
Participants randomized to active drug treatment tended to remain on active SHEP medication or on open-label antihypertensive drugs; thus, 89% were on active drug at year 3 and 90% at year 5. About 3% of the active treatment group received known active therapy because their blood pressure met escape criteria, and medication was stopped in 13% due to side effects. At the 5-year visit, 30% of participants in the active treatment group were receiving step 1, dose 1 medication only (chlorthalidone 12.5 mg/d); 16% were receiving Step 1, dose 2 medication only (chlorthalidone 25 mg/d); 11% were receiving Step 2, dose 1 medication (atenolol 25 mg/d); 12% were receiving step 2, dose 2 medication (atenolol 50 mg/d); 21% were receiving other active medication; and 9% were receiving no antihypertensive drug. Thus, at the end of the trial, almost half of those randomized to active drug were receiving step 1 drug only, and more than two thirds of the active drug participants were receiving protocol drugs only.

   Although the majority of participants randomized to placebo received no active antihypertensive medication throughout the trial, the percentage for whom active drug was prescribed increased from 13% at year 1 to 33% at year 3 and 44% at year 5. At some time during the trial, about 15% of placebo participants met the escape criteria (mostly due to DBP) and were prescribed active therapy; medication was stopped in 7% due to side effects.

Mean SBP and DBP by treatment group
Throughout the trial, the mean SBP of the active treatment group was consistently about 26 mmHg lower than its mean baseline value of 170 mmHg. For the placebo group, the mean SBP was consistently about 15 mmHg lower than at baseline. At various times during the trial, the SHEP goal SBP was reached by 65 to 72% of persons in the active treatment group but only by 32 to 40% of those in the placebo group.

   The mean DBP of the active treatment group was lower than its mean baseline value of 77 mmHg by about 9 mmHg; the mean DBP of the placebo group was lower than at baseline by 4 to 5 mmHg.

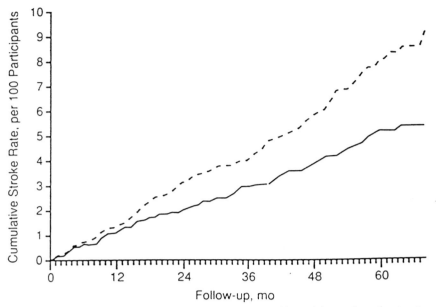

Figure 1. Cumulative fatal plus nonfatal stroke rate per 100 participants in active treatment (solid line) and placebo (broken line) groups during the Systolic Hypertension in the Elderly Program.

Total stroke incidence

With a mean follow-up of 4.5 years, incident stroke, the primary end point of the trial, was diagnosed in 103 persons in the active treatment group and 159 persons in the placebo group. Five-year cumulative stroke rates were 5.1 per 100 participants for the active treatment group and 7.9 per 100 participants for the placebo group. About 10% of strokes were fatal: 10 in the active treatment group and 14 in the placebo group.

Relative risk of developing a stroke during the trial for actively treated participants versus placebo participants was 0.64 (95% confidence interval (95% CI) was 0.50–0.82; $p = 0.0003$). The cumulative difference in the total stroke incidence rates increased progressively over the 5 years of the trial (The annual differences in cumulative rates were successively 0.2, 1.1, 1.2, 2.0 and 3.0 events per 100 participants, with rates being consistently lower in the active treatment group than in the placebo group). As shown in Figure 1, treatment was associated with no difference in stroke rates for 6 months, and with little difference for the next 6–9 months; thereafter, the differences in cumulative stroke incidence rates for the active treatment and placebo groups increased at an essentially constant rate. Active treatment reduced the 5-year risk of stroke by 28 events per 1000 actively treated participants.

Table 1.

	Total	SAH	IPH	LAC	CE	ATH	Ischemic Non Specific	Stroke Type Unknown
ACT	103	1	8	23	9	13	40	9
PLA	159	4	15	43	16	13	60	8

By age, sex, race, and baseline SBP

Stroke incidence was lower in active treatment than in placebo participants for all age groups, both sexes, and both races. Moreover, the favorable trend with active treatment was noted irrespective of baseline SBP.

Stroke subtype

The type of stroke was carefully studied by the SHEP Endpoint Committee which was blinded to treatment group [6]. Hemorrhagic strokes were of two types, with the diagnosis dependent on the location determined by brain imaging: subarachnoid (SAH) or intraparenchymal (IPH). Ischemic stroke types were: lacunar (LAC), diagnosed by either a clinical lacunar syndrome or by an appropriately located small deep lesion; cardioembolic (CE), based on a recognized cardiac source of embolism (e.g., atrial fibrillation); or atherosclerotic (ATH), when a noninvasive test or angiography demonstrated severe stenosis or occlusion of an appropriate artery. Table 1 compares stroke type in the active treatment (ACT) and placebo (PLA) groups. Thus, although the numbers were small, treatment seemed to approximately halve 4 of the 5 specifically diagnosed types of stroke; however, it had no apparent effect on atherosclerotic stroke [6].

Severity of observed strokes

Stroke severity was examined in three ways and at three different time intervals after the stroke had occurred [7]:

1. Deaths during the 30 days after the first stroke: 10 of 103 (9.7%) actively treated participants and 15 of 159 (9.4%) placebo participants with stroke died within 30 days.
2. Within 2 months of their first stroke, 4 participants in the active treatment group and 14 in the placebo group were placed in a nursing home.
3. Ordinary activities were examined at least 6 months after their first stroke for the 88 survivors (85%) in the active treatment group and for the 136 survivors (86%) in the placebo group. For the former there was a reduction of ordinary activities which averaged 0.8 days in the preceding two weeks. The comparable average reduction was 4.8 days for participants in the placebo group. Thus, strokes occurring in the placebo group were more severe than the smaller number of strokes occurring in the active treatment group [7].

Results by prior antihypertensive drug treatment
One of the two SHEP subgroup hypotheses was related to the expectation of a diminished effect of active treatment for participants who were already receiving antihypertensive medication at initial contact. The results did not indicate any such diminution. For the two-thirds of participants not receiving antihypertensive medication at initial contact, the relative risk of stroke for active treatment group compared with placebo group was 0.69 (95% CI, 0.51–0.95). For participants receiving antihypertensive medication at initial contact, the comparable relative risk for stroke was 0.57 (95% CI, 0.38–0.85). Thus, SHEP found a highly consistent decrease in strokes for the active treatment group, with no diminished effect in previously treated participants.

Cardiovascular events
The total number of cardiovascular events, both fatal and nonfatal, was 289 for active treatment and 414 for placebo participants, with a relative risk of 0.68 (95% CI, 0.58–0.79) and a 5-year absolute decrease of 55 events per 1000 participants. All coronary heart disease events, nonfatal plus fatal, numbered 140 for the active treatment group and 184 for the placebo group, with a relative risk of 0.75 (95% CI, 0.60–0.94) and a 5-year absolute benefit of 16 events per 1000 participants. As indicated in Table 2, these differences were statistically significant.

Baseline ECG abnormalities
The second a priori subgroup hypothesis was that the incidence of nonfatal myocardial infarction plus coronary death (including fatal myocardial infarction and sudden and rapid death) would be lower in participants without baseline ECG abnormalities than in those with abnormalities. For the 39% of patients free of baseline ECG abnormalities, the relative risk of cardiovascular disease events compared with placebo was 0.83 (95% CI, 0.53–1.29). For participants with baseline ECG abnormalities, the relative risk was 0.69 (95% CI, 0.50–0.94). Thus, the data do not support this subgroup hypothesis and suggest similar benefit from active treatment for both those with and without baseline ECG abnormalities.

Total and cause-specific mortality
The number of deaths was lower among active treatment participants than among placebo participants for mortality from all causes (213 versus 242 deaths), from total cardiovascular causes (90 versus 112 deaths), and from total coronary causes (59 versus 73 deaths) (range of relative risks, 0.80–0.87). None of these differences, however, was significant. In contrast, the number of deaths from neoplastic diseases, second only to cardiovascular disease as a cause of mortality for SHEP participants, was similar (77 deaths each) for the active treatment and placebo groups.

Table 2. Morbidity and mortality by cause and treatment group

	Number of events		Relative risk and (95% confidence interval)[a]
	Active therapy (n=2365)	Placebo group (n=2371)	
All events			
First stroke	103	159	0.64 (0.50–0.82)
Transient ischemic attack	62	82	0.75 (0.54–1.04)
Myocardial infarcation[b]	104	141	0.73 (0.57–0.94)
Coronary artery bypass & angioplasty	48	69	0.69 (0.48–0.998)
Left-ventricular failure	55	105	0.51 (0.37–0.71)
Renal dysfunction	8	13	0.61 (0.25–1.48)
Combined end-points			
All coronary heart disease[c]	140	184	0.75 (0.60–0.94)
All strokes & coronary heart disease	199	289	0.67 (0.56–0.81)
All cardiovascular disease[d]	289	414	0.68(0.58–0.79)
Number of fatal events			
Total deaths	213	242	0.87 (0.73–1.05)
Total cardiovascular	90	112	0.80 (0.61–1.05)
Stroke	10	14	0.71 (0.32–1.60)
Total coronary heart disease	59	73	0.80 (0.57–1.13)
Myocardial infarction	15	26	0.57 (0.30–1.08)
Sudden & rapid death (<24 h)	44	47	0.93 (0.62–1.40)
Left-ventricular failure	9	8	
Other	12	17	0.83 (0.47–1.49)
Total noncardiovascular	109	103	1.05 (0.80–1.38)
Neoplastic disease	77	77	0.99 (0.73–1.36)
Renal disease	2	2	
Infectious disease	11	8	
Accident, suicide, & homicide	5	5	
Other noncardiovascular	14	11	
Indeterminate cause	14	27	1.27 (0.58–2.79)

[a] Relative risk assessments were done for all types of events except those with fewer than 20 events and indeterminate cause of death.
[b] Nonfatal myocardial infarction (not including silent myocardial infarction) and coronary heart disease death
[c] Coronary heart disease includes myocardial infarction, sudden and rapid cardiac death, coronary artery bypass graft, and angioplasty.
[d] Cardiovascular disease includes coronary heart disease (vide supra), stroke, transient ischemic attack, aneurysm, and endarterectomy.

Hospitalizations and nursing home admissions
Hospitalizations for any reason occurred for 1027 active treatment partici-
pants (1976 admissions) and for 1086 placebo participants (2204 admissions).
This was not a significant difference.

Mental status
About 4% of the persons in both the active treatment and placebo groups
met questionnaire criteria for evaluation of possible dementia. More than
90% of the participants who met criteria completed a referral for further
diagnostic evaluation; the main reason for failure to achieve referral was
participant refusal. Thirty-seven participants receiving active treatment
(1.6%) and 44 receiving placebo (1.9%) had a diagnosis of dementia made
and subsequently confirmed by the Endpoint Committee which was blinded
to treatment group.

   During the trial, 14% of the persons in the active treatment group and
15% in the placebo group met the questionnaire criteria for evaluation of
possible depression. More than 75% of these participants completed a referral, and again the main reason for failure to achieve referral was participant
refusal. For 104 (4.4%) active treatment participants and 112 (4.7%) placebo
participants a definite diagnosis of depression was made.

   At baseline, 4.5% of the active treatment group and 5.7% of the placebo
group reported limitations in one or more of seven basic activities of daily
life. By the end of follow-up, 18.6% of the active treatment group and 20.1%
of the placebo group reported some decrease in their ability to accomplish
these activities ($p = 0.203$).

   Thus, there was no evidence of decreased mentation, undesirable mood
shifts, or changes in activities of daily living due to active antihypertensive
therapy.

Symptoms
At baseline, the total number of reported symptoms was similar in the active
and placebo treatment groups. During the entire course of the Trial 90.1%
of those on active therapy and 89.4% of those on placebo therapy complained
of troublesome or intolerable side effects at some time. Intolerable side
effects were reported by 28.1% of those assigned to active treatment and by
20.8% of those assigned to placebo.

   Persons on active therapy had significantly more faintness on standing
(22.2% versus 19.2%), cold or numb hands (17.3% versus 14.5%), excessive
thirst (8.2% versus 6.3%), loss of consciousness/passing out (4.4% versus
2.6%), and sexual dysfunction (8.1% versus 6.0%) than did those on placebo
therapy.

   Persons assigned to the placebo group had significantly more episodes of
rapid heart rate or irregular pulse (14.6% versus 12.0%), severe headaches
(15.8% versus 12.4%), and weakness/numbness on one side of the body
(5.8% versus 4.4%). The two groups did not differ with respect to chest pain,

shortness of breath, ankle swelling, falls or fractures, depression, nightmares, sleep problems, worry/anxiety, loss of appetite, nausea, skin rash, stuffy nose, joint pains, unsteadiness/imbalance, muscle weakness or cramping, indigestion, slow heart beat, memory/concentration problems, nocturia, or tiredness.

Blood chemistry

At baseline, the serum potassium averaged 4.5 mmol/l. After one year, it had decreased by an average of 0.4 mmol/l in the actively treated group and by 0.1 mmol/l in the placebo group. At some time during the trial, it fell below 3.2 mmol/l in 3.9% of the actively treated group and 0.8% of the placebo group.

For serum glucose, the average level at baseline was 6.0 mmol/l; after one year it had risen to 6.4 in the actively treated and 6.1 mmol/l in the placebo group, with 11.5% of the former and 9.7% of the latter having values greater than 11.1 mmol/l at some time during the trial.

For total serum cholesterol, the average level at baseline was 6.1 mmol/l; after one year it had risen to 6.3 mmol/l in the actively treated group, and it had not changed in the placebo group. At some time during the trial, 13.3% of the actively treated group and 11.1% of the placebo group had a value greater than 7.76 mmol/l.

Discussion

The SHEP is the first trial to test the efficacy of antihypertensive drug treatment in decreasing the incidence of the cardiovascular complications of ISH. The significant positive outcome on its primary endpoint of stroke unequivocally confirms the trend found in the SHEP pilot study [1]. The 36% reduction in stroke incidence is similar to that found in trials of drug therapy for diastolic hypertension, including the Hypertension Detection and Follow-up Program, the Medical Research Council trial, and 12 smaller trials combined [2]. Overall, these previous trials recorded a 42% reduction in stroke incidence (95% CI, 30%–54%). Findings from SHEP and other trials suggest that antihypertensive drug treatment is broadly effective, with similar reductions in the stroke rate for people with either diastolic hypertension or ISH.

Moreover, the SHEP decrease of 27% in incidence of nonfatal myocardial infarction plus coronary heart disease death for the active treatment group is similar to results of the Hypertension Detection and Follow-up Program and greater than those in other trials. Combined results of all diastolic hypertension trials indicate that a net decrease in blood pressure induced by active intervention was associated with a reduction of 14% (95% CI, 4%–24%) in incidence of major coronary events [3].

The positive SHEP outcome was achieved with minimum effective doses of antihypertensive drugs in a stepped-care regimen structured to achieve and maintain a goal blood pressure of at least 20 mmHg below baseline and below 160 mmHg, using 12.5 mg/d of chlorthalidone as the step 1 medication. High-level adherence to this regimen was maintained throughout the 5 years of the trial. During the trial, this regimen (plus the effects of regression to the mean and adaptation to clinic assessment) decreased the average SBP of the active treatment group about 26 mmHg below the pretreatment baseline level; the comparable decrease in SBP was 11 mmHg for the placebo group. The average DBP of the active treatment group was about 3–4 mmHg lower than the DBP of the placebo group. These data demonstrate an ability to achieve and sustain control of ISH in older persons with a low-dose, stepped-care drug regimen. This regimen was associated with infrequent adverse effects and no evidence of increase in dementia or depression.

It is a reasonable inference from the SHEP findings that middle-aged and older people with isolated or primarily systolic hypertension will benefit from such therapy. It also seems likely that those with less severe degrees of these conditions, particularly when other risk factors are present, will also benefit from treatment. Another reasonable implication from SHEP relates to the matter of preferred drug treatment regimens for any type of hypertension, in middle-aged as well as older people. A low-dose diuretic regimen is the initial treatment of choice for most hypertensive patients, based on demonstrated reduction in risk for major cardiovascular events, including coronary heart disease, and its safety, patient acceptance, and low cost.

In conclusion, SHEP demonstrated significant efficacy of active antihypertensive drug treatment in preventing stroke in persons aged 60 years and older with ISH. This result was achieved: (1) with use of stepped-care treatment, starting with low-dose chlorthalidone as the step 1 medication; (2) with the majority of participants assigned to active drug therapy being at or below the goal blood pressure; (3) with little increase in adverse effects; and (4) with no excess incidence of depression or dementia. Favorable findings were demonstrated for multiple secondary endpoints of the trial, including the incidence of major cardiac and cardiovascular events. These findings indicate a considerable potential for decreasing morbidity and disability by effective sustained drug treatment of ISH, given its prevalence and the high rates of cardiovascular diseases in those currently 60 years of age and older coupled with the rapid aging of our population.

References

1. Perry HM, Jr, Smith WM, McDonald RH et al. Morbidity and mortality in the Systolic Hypertension in the Elderly Program (SHEP) Pilot Study. Stroke 1989; **20**: 4–13.
2. Joint National Committee. The Fifth report of the Joint National Committee on detection, evaluation, and treatment of high blood pressure. Arch Intern Med. 1993; **153**: 154–83.
3. Collins R, Peto R, MacMahon S et al. Blood pressure, stroke and coronary heart disease

II: Short-term reductions in blood pressure; overview of randomized drug trials in their epidemiological context. Lancet 1990; **335**: 827–38.
4. SHEP Cooperative Research Group: Prevention of stroke by antihypertensive drug treatment in older persons with isolated systolic hypertension, Final results of the Systolic Hypertension in the Elderly Program (SHEP). JAMA 1991; **265**: 24; 3255.
5. Hulley SB, Furberg CD, Gurland B et al. The Systolic Hypertension in the Elderly Program (SHEP): Antihypertensive efficacy of chlorthalidone, Am J Cardiol 1985; **56**: 913.
6. The SHEP Cooperative Research Group: Prevention of Various Stroke Types by treatment of isolated systolic hypertension. Presented at the Second World Congress of Stroke, International Stroke Society, September 8–12, Washington, DC, 1992.
7. The SHEP Cooperative Research Group: The prevention of stroke by treatment of isolated systolic hypertension – strokes prevented are not mild. Presented at Second World Congress of Stroke, International Stroke Society, September 8–12, Washington, DC, 1992.
8. The SHEP Cooperative Research Group: Implications of the Systolic Hypertension in the Elderly Program, Hypertens 1993; **21**; 3: 335–43.

Index

Developments in Cardiovascular Medicine

28. B. Surawicz, C.P. Reddy and E.N. Prystowsky (eds.): *Tachycardias*. 1984
ISBN 0-89838-588-1

29. M.P. Spencer (ed.): *Cardiac Doppler Diagnosis*. Proceedings of a Symposium, held in Clearwater, Fla., U.S.A. (1983). 1983
ISBN 0-89838-591-1

30. H. Villarreal and M.P. Sambhi (eds.): *Topics in Pathophysiology of Hypertension*. 1984
ISBN 0-89838-595-4

31. F.H. Messerli (ed.): *Cardiovascular Disease in the Elderly*. 1984
Revised edition, 1988: see below under Volume 76

32. M.L. Simoons and J.H.C. Reiber (eds.): *Nuclear Imaging in Clinical Cardiology*. 1984
ISBN 0-89838-599-7

33. H.E.D.J. ter Keurs and J.J. Schipperheyn (eds.): *Cardiac Left Ventricular Hypertrophy*. 1983
ISBN 0-89838-612-8

34. N. Sperelakis (ed.): *Physiology and Pathology of the Heart*. 1984
Revised edition, 1988: see below under Volume 90

35. F.H. Messerli (ed.): *Kidney in Essential Hypertension*. Proceedings of a Course, held in New Orleans, La., U.S.A. (1983). 1984
ISBN 0-89838-616-0

36. M.P. Sambhi (ed.): *Fundamental Fault in Hypertension*. 1984   ISBN 0-89838-638-1

37. C. Marchesi (ed.): *Ambulatory Monitoring*. Cardiovascular System and Allied Applications. Proceedings of a Workshop, held in Pisa, Italy (1983). 1984
ISBN 0-89838-642-X

38. W. Kupper, R.N. MacAlpin and W. Bleifeld (eds.): *Coronary Tone in Ischemic Heart Disease*. 1984
ISBN 0-89838-646-2

39. N. Sperelakis and J.B. Caulfield (eds.): *Calcium Antagonists*. Mechanism of Action on Cardiac Muscle and Vascular Smooth Muscle. Proceedings of the 5th Annual Meeting of the American Section of the I.S.H.R., held in Hilton Head, S.C., U.S.A. (1983). 1984
ISBN 0-89838-655-1

40. Th. Godfraind, A.G. Herman and D. Wellens (eds.): *Calcium Entry Blockers in Cardiovascular and Cerebral Dysfunctions*. 1984   ISBN 0-89838-658-6

41. J. Morganroth and E.N. Moore (eds.): *Interventions in the Acute Phase of Myocardial Infarction*. Proceedings of the 4th Symposium on New Drugs and Devices, held in Philadelphia, Pa., U.S.A. (1983). 1984
ISBN 0-89838-659-4

42. F.L. Abel and W.H. Newman (eds.): *Functional Aspects of the Normal, Hypertrophied and Failing Heart*. Proceedings of the 5th Annual Meeting of the American Section of the I.S.H.R., held in Hilton Head, S.C., U.S.A. (1983). 1984
ISBN 0-89838-665-9

43. S. Sideman and R. Beyar (eds.): [3-D] *Simulation and Imaging of the Cardiac System*. State of the Heart. Proceedings of the International Henry Goldberg Workshop, held in Haifa, Israel (1984). 1985
ISBN 0-89838-687-X

44. E. van der Wall and K.I. Lie (eds.): *Recent Views on Hypertrophic Cardiomyopathy*. Proceedings of a Symposium, held in Groningen, The Netherlands (1984). 1985
ISBN 0-89838-694-2

45. R.E. Beamish, P.K. Singal and N.S. Dhalla (eds.), *Stress and Heart Disease*. Proceedings of a International Symposium, held in Winnipeg, Canada, 1984 (Vol. 1). 1985
ISBN 0-89838-709-4

46. R.E. Beamish, V. Panagia and N.S. Dhalla (eds.): *Pathogenesis of Stress-induced Heart Disease*. Proceedings of a International Symposium, held in Winnipeg, Canada, 1984 (Vol. 2). 1985
ISBN 0-89838-710-8

47. J. Morganroth and E.N. Moore (eds.): *Cardiac Arrhythmias*. New Therapeutic Drugs and Devices. Proceedings of the 5th Symposium on New Drugs and Devices, held in Philadelphia, Pa., U.S.A. (1984). 1985
ISBN 0-89838-716-7

48. P. Mathes (ed.): *Secondary Prevention in Coronary Artery Disease and Myocardial Infarction*. 1985
ISBN 0-89838-736-1

49. H.L. Stone and W.B. Weglicki (eds.): *Pathobiology of Cardiovascular Injury*. Proceedings of the 6th Annual Meeting of the American Section of the I.S.H.R., held in Oklahoma City, Okla., U.S.A. (1984). 1985
ISBN 0-89838-743-4

Developments in Cardiovascular Medicine

50. J. Meyer, R. Erbel and H.J. Rupprecht (eds.): *Improvement of Myocardial Perfusion.* Thrombolysis, Angioplasty, Bypass Surgery. Proceedings of a Symposium, held in Mainz, F.R.G. (1984). 1985   ISBN 0-89838-748-5
51. J.H.C. Reiber, P.W. Serruys and C.J. Slager (eds.): *Quantitative Coronary and Left Ventricular Cineangiography.* Methodology and Clinical Applications. 1986   ISBN 0-89838-760-4
52. R.H. Fagard and I.E. Bekaert (eds.): *Sports Cardiology.* Exercise in Health and Cardiovascular Disease. Proceedings from an International Conference, held in Knokke, Belgium (1985). 1986   ISBN 0-89838-782-5
53. J.H.C. Reiber and P.W. Serruys (eds.): *State of the Art in Quantitative Cornary Arteriography.* 1986   ISBN 0-89838-804-X
54. J. Roelandt (ed.): *Color Doppler Flow Imaging and Other Advances in Doppler Echocardiography.* 1986   ISBN 0-89838-806-6
55. E.E. van der Wall (ed.): *Noninvasive Imaging of Cardiac Metabolism.* Single Photon Scintigraphy, Positron Emission Tomography and Nuclear Magnetic Resonance. 1987   ISBN 0-89838-812-0
56. J. Liebman, R. Plonsey and Y. Rudy (eds.): *Pediatric and Fundamental Electrocardiography.* 1987   ISBN 0-89838-815-5
57. H.H. Hilger, V. Hombach and W.J. Rashkind (eds.), *Invasive Cardiovascular Therapy.* Proceedings of an International Symposium, held in Cologne, F.R.G. (1985). 1987   ISBN 0-89838-818-X
58. P.W. Serruys and G.T. Meester (eds.): *Coronary Angioplasty.* A Controlled Model for Ischemia. 1986   ISBN 0-89838-819-8
59. J.E. Tooke and L.H. Smaje (eds.): *Clinical Investigation of the Microcirculation.* Proceedings of an International Meeting, held in London, U.K. (1985). 1987   ISBN 0-89838-833-3
60. R.Th. van Dam and A. van Oosterom (eds.): *Electrocardiographic Body Surface Mapping.* Proceedings of the 3rd International Symposium on B.S.M., held in Nijmegen, The Netherlands (1985). 1986   ISBN 0-89838-834-1
61. M.P. Spencer (ed.): *Ultrasonic Diagnosis of Cerebrovascular Disease.* Doppler Techniques and Pulse Echo Imaging. 1987   ISBN 0-89838-836-8
62. M.J. Legato (ed.): *The Stressed Heart.* 1987   ISBN 0-89838-849-X
63. M.E. Safar (ed.): *Arterial and Venous Systems in Essential Hypertension.* With Assistance of G.M. London, A.Ch. Simon and Y.A. Weiss. 1987   ISBN 0-89838-857-0
64. J. Roelandt (ed.): *Digital Techniques in Echocardiography.* 1987   ISBN 0-89838-861-9
65. N.S. Dhalla, P.K. Singal and R.E. Beamish (eds.): *Pathology of Heart Disease.* Proceedings of the 8th Annual Meeting of the American Section of the I.S.H.R., held in Winnipeg, Canada, 1986 (Vol. 1). 1987   ISBN 0-89838-864-3
66. N.S. Dhalla, G.N. Pierce and R.E. Beamish (eds.): *Heart Function and Metabolism.* Proceedings of the 8th Annual Meeting of the American Section of the I.S.H.R., held in Winnipeg, Canada, 1986 (Vol. 2). 1987   ISBN 0-89838-865-1
67. N.S. Dhalla, I.R. Innes and R.E. Beamish (eds.): *Myocardial Ischemia.* Proceedings of a Satellite Symposium of the 30th International Physiological Congress, held in Winnipeg, Canada (1986). 1987   ISBN 0-89838-866-X
68. R.E. Beamish, V. Panagia and N.S. Dhalla (eds.): *Pharmacological Aspects of Heart Disease.* Proceedings of an International Symposium, held in Winnipeg, Canada (1986). 1987   ISBN 0-89838-867-8
69. H.E.D.J. ter Keurs and J.V. Tyberg (eds.): *Mechanics of the Circulation.* Proceedings of a Satellite Symposium of the 30th International Physiological Congress, held in Banff, Alberta, Canada (1986). 1987   ISBN 0-89838-870-8
70. S. Sideman and R. Beyar (eds.): *Activation, Metabolism and Perfusion of the Heart.* Simulation and Experimental Models. Proceedings of the 3rd Henry Goldberg Workshop, held in Piscataway, N.J., U.S.A. (1986). 1987   ISBN 0-89838-871-6

Developments in Cardiovascular Medicine

71. E. Aliot and R. Lazzara (eds.): *Ventricular Tachycardias.* From Mechanism to Therapy. 1987
ISBN 0-89838-881-3
72. A. Schneeweiss and G. Schettler: *Cardiovascular Drug Therapoy in the Elderly.* 1988
ISBN 0-89838-883-X
73. J.V. Chapman and A. Sgalambro (eds.): *Basic Concepts in Doppler Echocardiography.* Methods of Clinical Applications based on a Multi-modality Doppler Approach. 1987
ISBN 0-89838-888-0
74. S. Chien, J. Dormandy, E. Ernst and A. Matrai (eds.): *Clinical Hemorheology.* Applications in Cardiovascular and Hematological Disease, Diabetes, Surgery and Gynecology. 1987
ISBN 0-89838-807-4
75. J. Morganroth and E.N. Moore (eds.): *Congestive Heart Failure.* Proceedings of the 7th Annual Symposium on New Drugs and Devices, held in Philadelphia, Pa., U.S.A. (1986). 1987
ISBN 0-89838-955-0
76. F.H. Messerli (ed.): *Cardiovascular Disease in the Elderly.* 2nd ed. 1988
ISBN 0-89838-962-3
77. P.H. Heintzen and J.H. Bürsch (eds.): *Progress in Digital Angiocardiography.* 1988
ISBN 0-89838-965-8
78. M.M. Scheinman (ed.): *Catheter Ablation of Cardiac Arrhythmias.* Basic Bioelectrical Effects and Clinical Indications. 1988
ISBN 0-89838-967-4
79. J.A.E. Spaan, A.V.G. Bruschke and A.C. Gittenberger-De Groot (eds.): *Coronary Circulation.* From Basic Mechanisms to Clinical Implications. 1987
ISBN 0-89838-978-X
80. C. Visser, G. Kan and R.S. Meltzer (eds.): *Echocardiography in Coronary Artery Disease.* 1988
ISBN 0-89838-979-8
81. A. Bayés de Luna, A. Betriu and G. Permanyer (eds.): *Therapeutics in Cardiology.* 1988
ISBN 0-89838-981-X
82. D.M. Mirvis (ed.): *Body Surface Electrocardiographic Mapping.* 1988
ISBN 0-89838-983-6
83. M.A. Konstam and J.M. Isner (eds.): *The Right Ventricle.* 1988   ISBN 0-89838-987-9
84. C.T. Kappagoda and P.V. Greenwood (eds.): *Long-term Management of Patients after Myocardial Infarction.* 1988
ISBN 0-89838-352-8
85. W.H. Gaasch and H.J. Levine (eds.): *Chronic Aortic Regurgitation.* 1988
ISBN 0-89838-364-1
86. P.K. Singal (ed.): *Oxygen Radicals in the Pathophysiology of Heart Disease.* 1988
ISBN 0-89838-375-7
87. J.H.C. Reiber and P.W. Serruys (eds.): *New Developments in Quantitative Coronary Arteriography.* 1988
ISBN 0-89838-377-3
88. J. Morganroth and E.N. Moore (eds.): *Silent Myocardial Ischemia.* Proceedings of the 8th Annual Symposium on New Drugs and Devices (1987). 1988
ISBN 0-89838-380-3
89. H.E.D.J. ter Keurs and M.I.M. Noble (eds.): *Starling's Law of the Heart Revisted.* 1988
ISBN 0-89838-382-X
90. N. Sperelakis (ed.): *Physiology and Pathophysiology of the Heart.* Rev. ed. 1988
3rd, revised edition, 1994: see below under Volume 151
91. J.W. de Jong (ed.): *Myocardial Energy Metabolism.* 1988   ISBN 0-89838-394-3
92. V. Hombach, H.H. Hilger and H.L. Kennedy (eds.): *Electrocardiography and Cardiac Drug Therapy.* Proceedings of an International Symposium, held in Cologne, F.R.G. (1987). 1988
ISBN 0-89838-395-1
93. H. Iwata, J.B. Lombardini and T. Segawa (eds.): *Taurine and the Heart.* 1988
ISBN 0-89838-396-X
94. M.R. Rosen and Y. Palti (eds.): *Lethal Arrhythmias Resulting from Myocardial Ischemia and Infarction.* Proceedings of the 2nd Rappaport Symposium, held in Haifa, Israel (1988). 1988
ISBN 0-89838-401-X
95. M. Iwase and I. Sotobata: *Clinical Echocardiography.* With a Foreword by M.P. Spencer. 1989
ISBN 0-7923-0004-1

Developments in Cardiovascular Medicine

96. I. Cikes (ed.): *Echocardiography in Cardiac Interventions.* 1989
ISBN 0-7923-0088-2
97. E. Rapaport (ed.): *Early Interventions in Acute Myocardial Infarction.* 1989
ISBN 0-7923-0175-7
98. M.E. Safar and F. Fouad-Tarazi (eds.): *The Heart in Hypertension.* A Tribute to Robert C. Tarazi (1925-1986). 1989 ISBN 0-7923-0197-8
99. S. Meerbaum and R. Meltzer (eds.): *Myocardial Contrast Two-dimensional Echocardiography.* 1989 ISBN 0-7923-0205-2
100. J. Morganroth and E.N. Moore (eds.): *Risk/Benefit Analysis for the Use and Approval of Thrombolytic, Antiarrhythmic, and Hypolipidemic Agents.* Proceedings of the 9th Annual Symposium on New Drugs and Devices (1988). 1989 ISBN 0-7923-0294-X
101. P.W. Serruys, R. Simon and K.J. Beatt (eds.): *PTCA - An Investigational Tool and a Non-operative Treatment of Acute Ischemia.* 1990 ISBN 0-7923-0346-6
102. I.S. Anand, P.I. Wahi and N.S. Dhalla (eds.): *Pathophysiology and Pharmacology of Heart Disease.* 1989 ISBN 0-7923-0367-9
103. G.S. Abela (ed.): *Lasers in Cardiovascular Medicine and Surgery.* Fundamentals and Technique. 1990 ISBN 0-7923-0440-3
104. H.M. Piper (ed.): *Pathophysiology of Severe Ischemic Myocardial Injury.* 1990
ISBN 0-7923-0459-4
105. S.M. Teague (ed.): *Stress Doppler Echocardiography.* 1990 ISBN 0-7923-0499-3
106. P.R. Saxena, D.I. Wallis, W. Wouters and P. Bevan (eds.): *Cardiovascular Pharmacology of 5-Hydroxytryptamine.* Prospective Therapeutic Applications. 1990
ISBN 0-7923-0502-7
107. A.P. Shepherd and P.A. Öberg (eds.): *Laser-Doppler Blood Flowmetry.* 1990
ISBN 0-7923-0508-6
108. J. Soler-Soler, G. Permanyer-Miralda and J. Sagristà-Sauleda (eds.): *Pericardial Disease.* New Insights and Old Dilemmas. 1990 ISBN 0-7923-0510-8
109. J.P.M. Hamer: *Practical Echocardiography in the Adult.* With Doppler and Color-Doppler Flow Imaging. 1990 ISBN 0-7923-0670-8
110. A. Bayés de Luna, P. Brugada, J. Cosin Aguilar and F. Navarro Lopez (eds.): *Sudden Cardiac Death.* 1991 ISBN 0-7923-0716-X
111. E. Andries and R. Stroobandt (eds.): *Hemodynamics in Daily Practice.* 1991
ISBN 0-7923-0725-9
112. J. Morganroth and E.N. Moore (eds.): *Use and Approval of Antihypertensive Agents and Surrogate Endpoints for the Approval of Drugs affecting Antiarrhythmic Heart Failure and Hypolipidemia.* Proceedings of the 10th Annual Symposium on New Drugs and Devices (1989). 1990 ISBN 0-7923-0756-9
113. S. Iliceto, P. Rizzon and J.R.T.C. Roelandt (eds.): *Ultrasound in Coronary Artery Disease.* Present Role and Future Perspectives. 1990 ISBN 0-7923-0784-4
114. J.V. Chapman and G.R. Sutherland (eds.): *The Noninvasive Evaluation of Hemodynamics in Congenital Heart Disease.* Doppler Ultrasound Applications in the Adult and Pediatric Patient with Congenital Heart Disease. 1990
ISBN 0-7923-0836-0
115. G.T. Meester and F. Pinciroli (eds.): *Databases for Cardiology.* 1991
ISBN 0-7923-0886-7
116. B. Korecky and N.S. Dhalla (eds.): *Subcellular Basis of Contractile Failure.* 1990
ISBN 0-7923-0890-5
117. J.H.C. Reiber and P.W. Serruys (eds.): *Quantitative Coronary Arteriography.* 1991
ISBN 0-7923-0913-8
118. E. van der Wall and A. de Roos (eds.): *Magnetic Resonance Imaging in Coronary Artery Disease.* 1991 ISBN 0-7923-0940-5
119. V. Hombach, M. Kochs and A.J. Camm (eds.): *Interventional Techniques in Cardiovascular Medicine.* 1991 ISBN 0-7923-0956-1
120. R. Vos: *Drugs Looking for Diseases.* Innovative Drug Research and the Development of the Beta Blockers and the Calcium Antagonists. 1991 ISBN 0-7923-0968-5

Developments in Cardiovascular Medicine

Developments in Cardiovascular Medicine

Previous volumes are still available

KLUWER ACADEMIC PUBLISHERS – DORDRECHT / BOSTON / LONDON

**This book is to be returned on or before
the last date stamped below.**

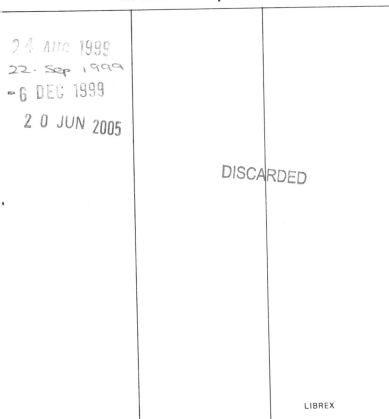

2 4 AUG 1999

22. Sep 1999

-6 DEC 1999

2 0 JUN 2005

DISCARDED

LIBREX

The Library, Ed & Trg Centre   KTW
Tunbridge Wells Hospital at Pembury
Tonbridge Rd, Pembury
Kent TN2 4QJ
01892 635884 and 635489

Prefix
MTW

0001475